A Diagnostic Atlas of Tumors of the Upper Aero-Digestive Tract

A Diagnostic Atlas of Tumors of the Upper Aero-Digestive Tract
A Transnasal Video Endoscopic Approach

Edited by

Tim Price

Consultant ENT Surgeon, Dorset County Hospital, NHS Foundation Trust, Dorset, UK

Paul Montgomery

Consultant ENT Surgeon, Bupa Cromwell Hospital, London, UK

Martin Birchall

Professor of Laryngology, UCL Ear Institute, London, UK
Consultant Laryngologist, Royal National Throat, Nose and Ear Hospital, London, UK

Patrick Gullane

Otolaryngologist-in-Chief, University Health Network, Toronto, Canada
Wharton Chair, Head and Neck Surgery, Princess Margaret Hospital, Toronto, Canada
Professor and Chair, Department of Otolaryngology-Head and Neck Surgery,
University of Toronto, Canada

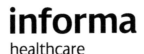

First published in 2012 by Informa Healthcare, 119 Farringdon Road, London EC1R 3DA, UK.

Simultaneously published in the USA by Informa Healthcare, 52 Vanderbilt Avenue, 7th Floor, New York, NY 10017, USA.

Informa Healthcare is a trading division of Informa UK Ltd. Registered Office: 37-41 Mortimer Street, London W1T 3JH, UK. Registered in England and Wales number 1072954.

A CIP record for this book is available from the British Library.

Library of Congress Cataloguing-in-Publication Data available on application

ISBN-13: 978-0-415-46630-1
eISBN: 978-1-84184-960-7

Orders may be sent to: Informa Healthcare, Sheepen Place, Colchester, Essex CO3 3LP, UK
Telephone: +44 (0)20 7017 6682
Email: Books@Informa.com
Website: http://informahealthcarebooks.com

For corporate sales please contact: CorporateBooksIHC@informa.com
For foreign rights please contact: RightsIHC@informa.com
For reprint permissions please contact: PermissionsIHC@informa.com

Typeset by Exeter Premedia Services Private Ltd, Chennai, India
Printed and bound in the United Kingdom

Dedication

I would like to dedicate this book to my wife, Susan and our children Leah, Abigail, and Hannah for their patience, support, and the sacrifice of family time. It is also dedicated to my parents for their love and support over the years. Thank you.

TP

I would like to dedicate this book to my children Isabelle, Harry, and Jemima for their sacrifice of family time and to my family, friends, and colleagues for their support.

PM

Contents

Contributors   ix
Foreword   x
Preface   xi
Video Clips   xii

SECTION 1: AN OVERVIEW

1.1 **An introduction to transnasal laryngoesophagoscopy**   1
Tim Price

1.2 **The technique: General and biopsy of lesions**   4
Tim Price and Tim Bradnam

1.3 **The patient's experience**   6
Alok Sharma

SECTION 2: PREMALIGANT DISORDERS AND MALIGNANT TUMORS

2.1 **Nasal cavity and paranasal sinuses**   8
Holger Sudhoff

2.2 **Nasopharynx**   13
Holger Sudhoff

2.3 **Oral cavity**   18
Richard C. W. James

2.4 **Oropharynx**

    2.4.1 **Oropharynx tumors**   23
    Tom Wilson

    2.4.2 **Tonsil tumors**   26
    Hemi Patel

    2.4.3 **Base of tongue tumors**   29
    Tim Price

2.5 **Larynx**

    2.5.1 **Supraglottic tumors**   32
    Mike Thomas

    2.5.2 **Glottic tumors**   35
    Mike Thomas and Tim Price

    2.5.3 **Subglottic tumors**   38
    Mike Thomas

2.6 Hypopharynx

    2.6.1 Hypopharynx tumors   40
    Tom Wilson

    2.6.2 Pyriform fossa tumors   42
    Hemi Patel

    2.6.3 Post cricoid tumors   45
    Wyn Parry

2.7 Esophageal tumors   48
Wyn Parry and Tim Price

2.8 Tracheal tumors   51
Wyn Parry

2.9 Tumors of the thyroid   54
Don J. Premachandra

SECTION 3: BENIGN TUMORS

3.1 Benign nasopharyngeal tumors   57
Hemi Patel

3.2 Oropharynx and parapharyngeal tumors

    3.2.1 Oropharynx tumors   60
    Tom Wilson

    3.2.2 Benign parapharyngeal tumors affecting the tonsils   63
    Hemi Patel

3.3 Larynx

    3.3.1 Supraglottis   66
    Mike Thomas

    3.3.2 Glottis   71
    Mike Thomas

    3.3.3 Subglottis   74
    Mike Thomas

SECTION 4: TREATMENT OPTIONS USING TNLE

4.1 Endolaryngeal laser surgery using TNLE   76
Tim Price

4.2 Direct phonoplasty   78
Alok Sharma

4.3 TNLE and tracheoesophageal puncture   80
James Snelling

SECTION 5: POST-TREATMENT MONITORING AND COMPLICATIONS

Section 5A: Surgical

5.1   **Total laryngectomy: Primary and flap repair**   82
       Animesh J. Patel and Jonothan J. Clibbon

5.2   **Flap monitoring**   86
       Animesh J. Patel and Jonothan J. Clibbon

5.3   **Flap necrosis and postoperative fistula**   89
       Jonothan J. Clibbon and Animesh J. Patel

5.4   **Surgical voice restoration**   91
       Gill Faley, Karyn Stewart-Dodd, and Sue Trim

Section 5B: Chemoradiation

5.5   **Radiation and chemoradiation in head and neck cancer**   94
       Craig Martin

Index   99

Contributors

Martin A. Birchall
University College and Royal National Throat Nose and Ear Hospital, London, UK

Tim Bradnam
Norfolk and Waveney Head and Neck Centre, Norfolk and Norwich University Hospitals NHS Foundation Trust, Norwich, UK

Jonothan J. Clibbon
Norfolk and Norwich University Hospitals NHS Foundation Trust, Norwich, UK

Gill Faley
Rehab Department, Dorset County Hospital, Dorchester, UK

Patrick Gullane
University Health Network, Toronto, Canada
Head and Neck Surgery, Princess Margaret Hospital, Toronto, Canada
Department of Otolaryngology-Head and Neck Surgery, University of Toronto, Canada

Richard C. W. James
Norfolk and Norwich University Hospitals NHS Foundation Trust, Norwich, UK

Matthew Lofthouse
Norfolk and Norwich University Hospitals NHS Foundation Trust, Norwich, UK

Craig Martin
Norfolk and Norfolk University Hospitals NHS Foundation Trust, Norwich, UK

Paul Montgomery
Bupa Cromwell Hospital, London, UK

Wyn Parry
Norfolk and Norwich University Hospitals NHS Foundation Trust, Norwich, UK
University of East Anglia School of Medicine, Norwich, UK

Animesh J. Patel
Norfolk and Norwich University Hospitals NHS Foundation Trust, Norwich, UK

Hemi Patel
Royal Darwin Hospital, Northern Territory, Darwin, Australia

Don J. Premachandra
James Paget and Norfolk and Norwich University Hospitals, Great Yarmouth, UK

Tim Price
Dorset County Hospital, Dorchester, UK

Alok Sharma
Royal Hospital for Sick Children, Edinburgh, UK

James Snelling
John Radcliffe Hospital, Oxford, UK

Karyn Stewart-Dodd
Rehabilitation Department, Dorset County Hospital, Dorchester, UK

Holger Sudhoff
Department of Otolaryngology, Head and Neck Surgery, Bielefeld Academic Teaching Hospital, Bielefeld, Germany

Mike Thomas
Gloucestershire Hospitals NHS Foundation Trust, Gloucestershire, UK

Sue Trim
Dorset County Hospital, Dorchester, UK

Paddy Wilson
Norfolk and Norwich University Hospitals NHS Foundation Trust, Norwich, UK

Tom Wilson
Leeds Teaching Hospitals NHS Trust, Yorkshire, UK

Foreword

Laryngology is the field of surgery that assesses and manages those with throat, voice, and swallowing disorders. Although dating back to the early nineteenth century, it has taken a back seat in certain things to other subspecialties of otolaryngology (ear, nose, and throat surgery) for many decades. However, the last fifteen years has seen a startling uplift in interest, research, training, and technology in this field. One result is that, in many otolaryngology departments in the United States, laryngologists have the highest patient throughput and even in some cases bring in the highest income of all ENT subspecialists. In parallel, there is an increasing recognition that the diagnosis and management of swallowing and other esophageal problems in particular have lagged well behind advances in other fields. This is despite the population impact and fundamental effect that dysphagia exerts on the quality of life.

This too is now being corrected, by an upsurge in research into diagnosis, treatments, and technology. Technology itself has advanced apace. The advent of progressively higher-resolution distal chip cameras and processors among other technical improvements has now led to the development of a range of transnasal esophagoscopes. So fundamental has the effect of these instruments been on laryngology and more generally, on otolaryngology in recent years, that we felt strongly that the knowledge of the reach and precision of transnasal esophagoscopes should be far more widespread.

To achieve this goal, as well as to assist in training programs, we conceived this book. We hope it will provide you with a view through the window into esophageal anatomy, physiology, and pathology that this wonderful device affords. The device has a smooth learning curve for those starting out with transnasal esophagoscopy anew and will improve their diagnostic acumen. It is clear to us that the technology has much further to go and that with it the range of diagnostic and therapeutic interventions available to the laryngologist will continue to expand. Thus, this book may be considered a starting point in many ways, but one which we hope will educate as well as fascinate in equal measure.

Martin A. Birchall, MD (Cantab), FRCS, F Med Sci,
Professor of Laryngology, University College London
Consultant in Otolaryngology, Royal National Throat,
Nose and Ear Hospital, London, UK

Preface

Over the past 15–20 years we have experienced a significant renaissance in our understanding, diagnostic techniques and management of tumors about the head and neck. During the plan for the development of the contents of this atlas it was felt that not only should it provide a comprehensive overview of the common presentations and diagnostic tools available but also select contributors with an experienced understanding of each of the subsites. The authors have been carefully chosen and represent different geographic regions so that a global perspective is obtained. Our appreciation and thanks to all the contributors for providing a remarkable product. As editors we are all familiar with the challenges of a multi-authored book.

The atlas is unique in its design and format. The objective is to provide the reader with an overview of benign and malignant tumors of the upper aero-digestive tract and to employ the current-day approaches using new technology. This practical atlas is intended for surgeons in training, those who are already in practice and as a resource for medical students and those in other specialties.

The atlas is divided into five sections.

SECTION ONE
This section contains a very practical overview that details the advantages and pitfalls in transnasal laryngoesophagoscopy. The chapters within this section are very informative and help the readers understand the challenges of the diagnostic approach and the techniques that minimize patients' discomfort.

SECTION TWO
This section focuses on the analysis and current treatment of both benign and malignant cancers of the nasopharynx, nose/sinuses, oral cavity, oropharynx, larynx, hypopharynx, trachea, esophagus, and thyroid. The choice of treatment and the options and limitations are dealt with in a very succinct and clear manner. The nuances and philosophies are very cleverly discussed leaving the reader with a thorough understanding of the present day choices.

SECTIONS THREE AND FOUR
These are designed to navigate the most challenging area; however, the addition of well-illustrated descriptions of case examples in each subsite makes these two sections very educational.

SECTION FIVE
This is a potpourri of ablative techniques, reconstructive options, rehabilitation, and finally, the current role of chemo/radiation. The chapters are very comprehensive and attempt to introduce the novice to the limitations and complications of Head and Neck Surgery and in addition, can be of immense benefit as a reference to the practitioners.

This atlas is the most important and timely overview, in our present knowledge, of both the diagnostic and therapeutic techniques available in present day practice to help enhance the management and outcome of patients with Head and Neck Neoplasms. It is hoped that our readers will benefit from the information contained in this atlas and that its contents will help to further enhance the quality of patient care and stimulate younger investigators to be innovative.

Patrick Gullane, CM, MB, FRCSC, FACS,
***Hon* FRACS, *Hon* FRCS**
Otolaryngologist-in-Chief, University Health Network
Wharton Chair, Head and Neck Surgery,
Princess Margaret Hospital Professor and Chair,
Department of Otolaryngology-Head and Neck Surgery
University of Toronto, Toronto, Canada

Acknowledgments

I thank Paul Montgomery for giving me the opportunity and the material to edit and write this book. Thanks are also to Alok Sharma for putting the video clips together. My thanks also go to Amber Thomas, Associate Managing Editor, for her help and encouragement in putting the book together.

Finally I would like to thank all those who contributed chapters and photographs; we got there in the end!

TP

Video Clips

The 13 video clips listed below and designated in the text by the video icon shown here are available for viewing at our website: http://www.informahealthcare.com.

To access the video clips, you will need to first register at our website where, upon completion of the registration process, you will have the necessary login details. If you have previously registered, there is no need to register again.

After you have completed the registration procedure, please type the following link in your web browser: http://www.informahealthcare.com/videos/9780415466301

The opening page will request your login details and, after signing in, the video clips will be available for viewing.

1. Technique of TNLE.

2. A pharyngeal pouch.

3. Removal of an ingested foreign body under local anesthetic.

4. Plum stone impacted at the gastroesophageal junction.

5. Demonstration of the technique of TNLE with an examination of the larynx.

6. Postnasal space lesion.

7. Biopsy of the vocal cord.

8. Biopsies of the right vocal cord.

9. Biopsy of a subglottic lesion.

10. Bilateral laryngoceles.

11. Endolaryngeal laser surgery.

12. Direct phonoplasty.

13. Secondary tracheoesophageal puncture.

1.1 An introduction to transnasal laryngoesophagoscopy
Tim Price

Transnasal flexible endoscopy, using fiberoptic instruments to examine the nose and larynx, is a long-established method, described originally in 1968. Recent advances in flexible endoscopic digital technology and miniaturization by the Pentax Corporation (Slough, U.K.) and improved local anesthetic techniques to both the nose and the larynx have led to the development of the transnasal laryngoesophagoscope (TNLE): The Pentax 80K Series Digital Video Endoscope (EE 1580K) (Figs. 1.1.1 & 1.1.2).

This is a 5.1-mm diameter flexible endoscope. It incorporates a high-resolution color Charge Coupled Device image sensor (CCD) chip in its tip, allowing full screen images of high definition to be viewed on the monitor. The high-definition digital video recording and playback permits a 43-msec, frame-by-frame analysis of high-quality images with no distortion. The latest recorders allow 30-msec recordings, capturing even more details. This is critically important when viewing the postcricoid area and the upper esophageal sphincter area which only opens momentarily when the patient swallows and is not easily visible in real time. This analysis is also enhanced by the reviewing of multiple swallowing events.

Suction, irrigation, and insufflation are possible with the TNLE and this assists in the examination of this difficult area (Video 1). It is now possible to study the postcricoid area in greater detail than ever before and in the outpatient department under local anesthesia (Fig. 1.1.3). Postcricoid webs are easily seen (Fig. 1.1.4).

Esophageal pouches, which are closely related to the postcricoid area and notoriously difficult to examine, are easily seen and assessed (Video 2). The new technology allows an incredibly clear view to be obtained thanks to the insufflation. Residual saliva and food debris in the pouch can be flushed out or suctioned out, allowing a detailed assessment of the pouch mucosa (Figs. 1.1.5–1.1.7). This therefore negates the need for a barium swallow and rigid esophagoscopy for diagnostic purposes.

There is a 2-mm instrument channel through which a variety of reusable endoscopic instruments can be used. The Pentax Biopsy Forceps (KW1811S) (Slough, U.K.) allows an accurate biopsy of any mucosal lesion (Fig. 1.1.8). The Pentax ENT Flex Needle (Slough, U.K.) (Fig. 1.1.9) allows for the injection of collagen for medialization of a paralyzed vocal cord (chap. 4.2).

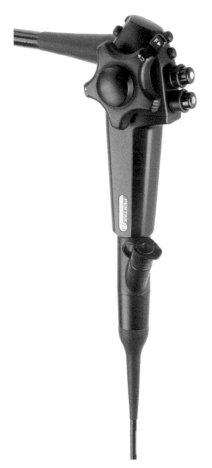

Figure 1.1.1 TNLE Scope (Pentax). Yellow button is for suction. Green button is for insufflation. The working channel is a little further down the hand piece.

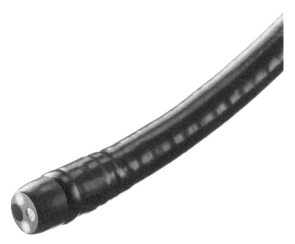

Figure 1.1.2 The distal end of the scope (Pentax) showing the working channel, light source, and camera lens.

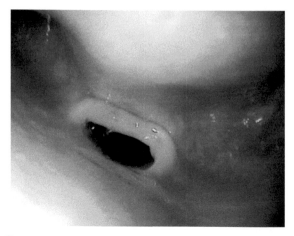

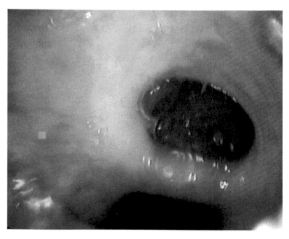

Figure 1.1.3 Postcricoid area, on a 43-msec frame-by-frame analysis, during swallowing. The posterior pharyngeal mucosa is seen inferiorly; the mucosa covering the posterior surface of the cricoid cartilage superiorly and the apices of the left and right piriform fossa on either side. The cricopharyngeal ring (upper esophageal sphincter) is seen beginning to open up in the center of the picture.

Figure 1.1.5 The pharyngeal pouch. The esophageal lumen is seen inferiorly and the posterior laryngeal surface superiorly. The prominent cricoid bar is seen centrally with the pouch above it filled with saliva and debris.

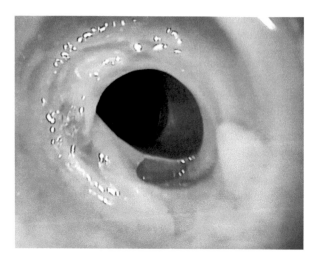

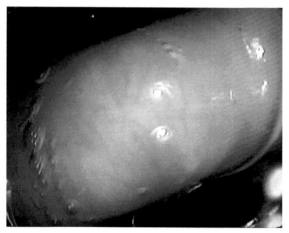

Figure 1.1.4 Postcricoid web.

Figure 1.1.6 The mucosa of the pouch "bar" can be examined in detail.

Virtually all patients referred to ENT outpatients who would normally be examined with an endoscope (flexible or rigid) are suitable for examination with the TNLE. TNLE can be performed under local anesthesia, without sedation, in a procedure room of the outpatients department, the day-surgery unit, or in the main theater suite. The chapters that follow illustrate how TNLE allows the surgeon to perform a variety of diagnostic and therapeutic procedures on the larynx, pharynx, and esophagus within these settings.

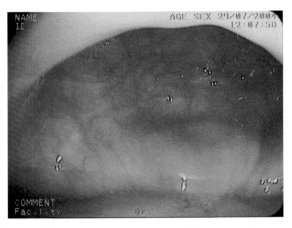

Figure 1.1.7 The pouch can be suctioned clear of the debris and the mucosa inspected for any lesions.

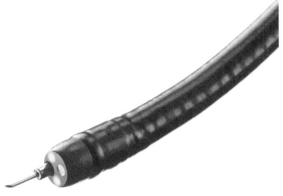

Figure 1.1.9 A 23-gauge needle (Pentax) that is fed through the operating port.

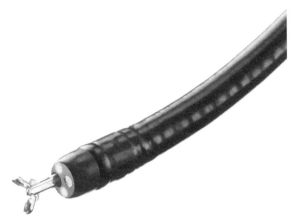

Figure 1.1.8 A biopsy forceps (Pentax) that is fed through the operating port.

1.2 The technique: General and biopsy of lesions
Tim Price and Tim Bradnam

LOCATION

Transnasal laryngoesophagoscopy (TNLE) is performed under local anesthesia without intravenous sedation (Video 1). It can therefore be safely performed in a procedure room in the outpatients department. If specialized facilities are needed for example, for laser surgery, it is performed in an operating theater.

LOCAL ANESTHESIA

The nose is first prepared with two sprays of lignocaine hydrochloride (5%)/ phenylephrine (0.5%) aerosol solution applied to each nostril; and 3 ml of lignocaine gel (containing 2% lignocaine) is then applied to both the anterior nares. The oropharynx is then sprayed with a further two sprays of lignocaine (10%) aerosol solution via the mouth. The remaining 4 ml of lignocaine gel is used as a lubricant on the endoscope itself, providing further topical analgesia for the endoscopy.

Depending on the procedure, the larynx may be further anesthetized, under direct vision, with up to 2 ml of 4% lignocaine. The authors have found that less than 0.5 ml is usually sufficient (Fig. 1.2.1 & Fig. 4.1.1 in chap. 4.1). This is delivered directly to the vocal cords via an epidural catheter (Portex® 16-gauge Ref 100/382/116, Smiths Medical ASD, Inc, Keene, NH03431, USA) that is passed down the instrument channel. A total dose of 350 mg of lignocaine is given which is about half of the total topical dose that can be administered to a 70-kg man (Table. 1.2.1).

POSITION

Our technique requires the patient to be sitting sideways on a treatment couch, facing the endoscopist. If the patient were to become unwell, they may safely be laid on the couch for resuscitation. The endoscope stack is positioned behind the patient in clear view of the endoscopist (Fig. 1.2.2).

PROCEDURE

The endoscope is passed transnasally allowing a view of the nasal cavity, postnasal space, base of the tongue, pharynx, larynx and both pyriform fossae. The patient is then instructed to swallow and the scope is advanced into the hypopharynx and esophagus, down to the gastroesophageal junction. The mucosal surface can

Table 1.2.1 Total Dose of Local Anesthesia Given to Each Patient

	Lignocaine (mg)
4 sprays lignocaine (5%)/ phenylephrine (0.5%) to nose	30
6 ml Instagel (lignocaine 2%) to nose	120
5 ml Instagel (lignocaine 2%) on endoscope	100
2 sprays lignocaine (10%) to mouth/oropharynx	20
2 ml lignocaine (4%) sprayed onto larynx	80
Total topical dose	**350**

Figure 1.2.1 Application of a local anesthetic via an epidural catheter to a paralyzed left vocal cord.

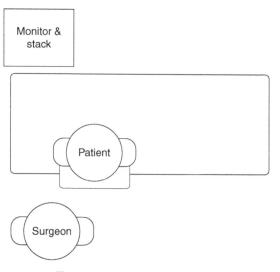

Figure 1.2.2 Layout of a procedure room.

be carefully inspected both on the way down the esophagus and again while withdrawing the scope. A biopsy or therapeutic procedure can be performed during this initial assessment.

A diagnosis is usually therefore possible and the recording is viewed with the patient. This enables them to understand what the problem is and to gain a better understanding of what we as surgeons need to do to help. Those that have a negative endoscopy are also greatly reassured because of the psychological benefit of having had visual re-enforcement that there is no pathology present to worry about.

RECOVERY

Patients are kept nil by mouth until the effects of the local anesthetic have worn off. In practice this means that patients are observed for 1–2 hours before discharge.

1.3 The patient's experience
Alok Sharma

Transnasal laryngoesophagoscopy (TNLE) is a safe and well-tolerated technique. It is well accepted by patients as it causes little discomfort and compares favorably with other endoscopic techniques.

PAIN SCORES

Using a simple visual analogue scale of 0–10, the patients' pain experience was evaluated. The 0 point indicated "no discomfort" and on the far right, 10 indicated "worst pain ever."

The patients were asked about nasal pain, throat pain, chest pain, stomach bloating, feeling to retch or vomit, a feeling of nausea or sickness, and overall discomfort during TNLE.

The majority of the patients recorded a very low visual analog score for a global evaluation of pain and discomfort. The mean and median pain scores were below 1 out of 10 for all evaluated discomforts (Table 1.3.1).

The procedure appears to cause little nasal or throat pain, with mean scores <1 (0.7 and 0.6 respectively), and median scores of <1 (0.4 and 0.3 respectively). The higher mean scores were observed by one individual finding this part of the procedure uncomfortable, with scores of 6.8 and 4.1; however, the majority had little discomfort which is reflected in the very low median scores and seen in the histograms (Fig. 1.3.1).

There appears to be little chest pain, caused by any esophageal discomfort, reported. The mean chest pain score was <1 (0.4) and the median score <1 (0.5).

TNLE did cause slight discomfort with feelings of bloating and retching in some individuals, with a mean score <1 (0.8 and 0.9 respectively) and a median score <1 (0.3 and 0.3 respectively). The histograms also demonstrate the tolerance by the majority (Fig. 1.3.1). Patients for whom more insufflation was required complained more of this discomfort.

TNLE does not appear to cause significant feelings of sickness or nausea, with low scores having a mean of <1 (0.4) and median of only <1 (0.1) (Table 1.3.1).

Table 1.3.1 Pain Scores

	Mean Score	Median Score	Min Score	Max. Score
Nasal pain/discomfort	0.724	0.4	0	6.8
Throat pain/discomfort	0.588	0.3	0	4.1
Chest pain/discomfort	0.444	0.5	0	5.7
Stomach bloating	0.824	0.3	0	5.2
Feeling to retch	0.982	0.3	0	5.1
Feeling of sickness	0.43	0.15	0	3
Overall discomfort	0.924	0.8	0	5.4

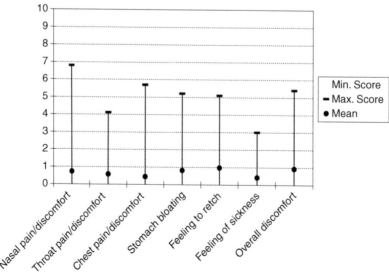

Figure 1.3.1 Distribution of pain scores. *Source*: Sharma A, Price T, Mierzwa K, et al. Transnasal flexible laryngo-oesophagoscopy: an evaluation of the patient's experience. The Journal of Laryngology & Otology 2006; 120(1): 24–31.

The overall discomfort score was again less than 1, with a mean score of <1 (0.9) and a median of <1 (0.8) (Table 1.3.1).

COMPLICATIONS

TNLE does not appear to have any major complications. Minor epistaxis caused by simple nasal trauma and easily controlled by pressure appears to occur in less than 2% of patients. Similar series have described syncope, but this has not been the experience of the authors.

TNLE VS. OTHER ENDOSCOPIC TECHNIQUES

The data reported here suggest the technique is well tolerated causing little overall discomfort in patients and compares favorably with other studies on pain associated with simple flexible endoscopy. The TNLE mean overall pain scores are <1, despite it being a larger diameter scope and used for a more extensive application during the procedure.

It is difficult to compare directly as other studies in endoscopy have used variable visual analog scale scores. However, TNLE compares favourably with simple flexible nasolaryngoscopy and esophagogastroduodenoscopy (both per oral and transnasal).

LOCAL ANESTHESIA IN TNLE

A key factor in the low pain scores of TNLE and good patient acceptance is the use of a local anesthetic. No sedation is required by the patient during TNLE.

2.1 Nasal cavity and paranasal sinuses
Holger Sudhoff

PRESENTATION

Malignant tumors of the nasal cavity or the paranasal sinuses are rare and present usually at an advanced stage due to the lack of early clinical symptoms. Symptoms are numerous and include headaches or pain in the sinus areas, blocked sinuses, rhinorrhea, and epistaxis; tooth pain in the maxilla, or dentures that no longer fit because of lumps in the hard palate/roof of the mouth; facial numbness, paresthesia, progressive pain, and facial asymmetry may occur; swelling and closure of the eyes with proptosis and associated blurred vision, double vision (diplopia) or visual loss. Otalgia is a further symptom. The average delay between the onset of symptoms and final diagnosis is 3–18 months.

ETIOLOGY AND HISTOLOGY

The most common malignant neoplasm of the nasal cavity and paranasal sinuses is squamous cell carcinoma (SCC), occurring in 70–80% of all cases (Fig. 2.1.1A–C). Regional

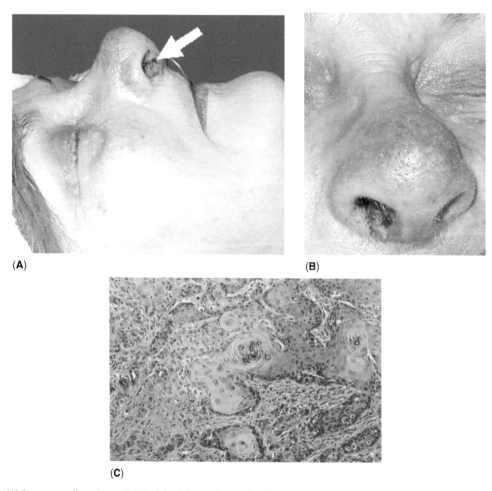

(A)

(B)

(C)

Figure 2.1.1 (A) Squamous cell carcinoma (SCC) of the right anterior nasal cavity in a 64-year-old female patient, with no obvious risk factors (arrow). After surgical removal of the tumor nasal reconstruction was achieved by covering a rib-cartilage framework with a forehead flap. (B) AP view of the SCC originating from the right nasal septum. (C) Histopathologic image illustrating a well-differentiated SCC in a high power view.

node involvement from primary SCC of the paranasal sinuses occurs in about 15% of all cases and distant metastases occur in approximately 9% of all cases. The etiology of tumors of the nasal cavity and paranasal sinuses is unknown but some clinical data indicate that smoking and various industrial exposures may be causative. Risk factors include the exposure to nickel, chromium, mustard gas, isopropyl alcohol, and radium.

In addition there is an association with inverted papillomas and SCC. Inverted papillomas are benign, locally aggressive sinonasal tumors with high rates of recurrence (chap. 3.1). The risk of malignant transformation in these tumors varies widely, ranging from 2–56%. Most surgeons therefore advocate radical surgical removal of them and a close follow-up to detect early recurrence.

Adenocarcinomas arising from the ethmoid or maxillary sinuses are frequently associated with exposure to industrial wood dust in hardwood and shoe industry workers (Fig. 2.1.2). Other malignant tumors of the paranasal sinuses that occur less frequently are adenoid cystic carcinoma (Figs. 2.1.3–2.1.6), mucoepidermoid carcinoma, malignant mixed tumor, adenocarcinoma, melanoma (Figs.2.1.7 & 2.1.8), esthesioneuroblastoma (Fig. 2.1.9), malignant nerve sheath tumor, lymphoma, fibrosarcoma, osteosarcoma, and chondrosarcoma. These tumors grow within the bony confines of the paranasal sinuses and often are asymptomatic until they erode or invade adjacent structures. Commonly, paranasal sinus tumors are slow growing with a low tendency to metastasize locally, regionally, or distally. Adenoid cystic carcinomas are notorious for local recurrence and distant

metastasis because of perineural invasion. The most common malignant neoplasm arising elsewhere and metastasizing to the paranasal sinuses is hypernephroma. Other metastatic lesions include undifferentiated tumors arising from the lungs, breasts, prostate, and pancreas.

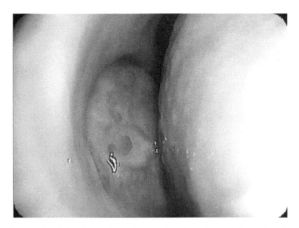

Figure 2.1.3 Adenoid cystic carcinoma of the lateral wall right nasal cavity.

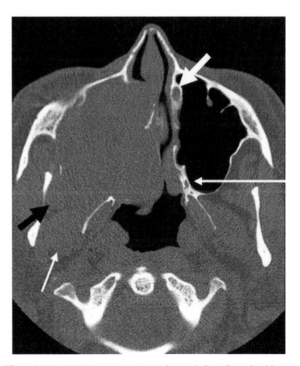

Figure 2.1.4 Axial CT scan post contrast; bone windows through midmaxillary antrum. The Adenoid cystic carcinoma extends into the nasal cavity and masticator space (black arrow). Note the involvement of the greater and lesser palatine foramina and the nasolacrimal duct. Normal left palatine foramina (long white arrow). Normal left nasolacrimal duct (thick white arrow). Lateral pterygoid muscle (short white arrow).

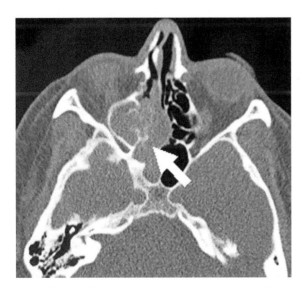

Figure 2.1.2 Axial CT scan at the level of orbits showing a right-sided adenocarcinoma infiltrating the posterior septum and right orbit in a 55-year-old cabinet maker (white arrow). Surgery was performed via midfacial degloving with postoperative intensity-modulated radiation therapy.

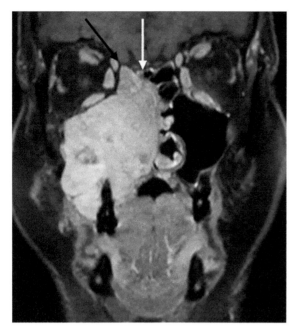

Figure 2.1.5 Adenoid cystic carcinoma centered on the right maxillary antrum. Coronal fat saturated T1 post contrast. Lesion extends up to cribriform plate (white arrow) but no evidence of extension into the cranial cavity. Note that high signal secretions in an adjacent ethmoid air cell (black arrow) are indistinguishable from the tumor on the fat saturation postcontrast images. There is a wide arc of contact with the orbit but no definite invasion.

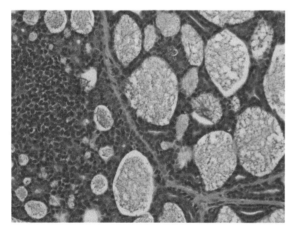

Figure 2.1.6 A cribriform adenoid cystic carcinoma characterized by nests of cells with cylindromatous microcystic spaces filled with mucoid material.

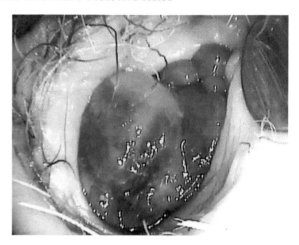

Figure 2.1.7 A malignant melanoma of the right nostril.

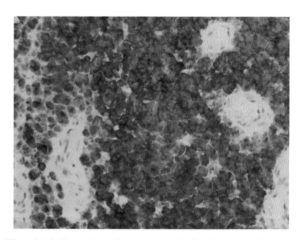

Figure 2.1.8 Sheets of densely packed, angulated melanocytes with prominent nuclei and positive staining with Melan-A in keeping with mucosal melanoma.

EPIDEMIOLOGY

Malignant tumors of the nasal cavity and paranasal sinuses constitute less than 1% of all malignancies in the body and about 3% of all head and neck cancers. The frequency among men is twice that of women. The annual incidence in a European population was found to be 1.7 cases per 100,000 persons. In the United States and Israel, the annual incidence is less than 1 case per 100,000. SCC is the most common tumor (Fig. 2.1.1C). Approximately 80% of these tumors arise in the maxillary sinus, while about 20% occur in the ethmoid sinuses; less than 1% of these arise from the frontal and sphenoid sinuses and in the nose. Adenocarcinomas make up 4–8% of all sinonasal cancer. They originate most commonly at the ethmoids and nasal cavity, and are locally aggressive. Adenocarcinoma of the sinus may also resemble a moderately differentiated colon adenocarcinoma. Adenoid cystic carcinoma accounts for 6% of the sinonasal tract cancer. Mucoepidermoid and neuroendocrine carcinomas are extremely rare in the sinonasal tract.

IMAGING

Preferred examinations include the following: clinical examination of the neck, cranial nerves examination, and rigid or fiberoptic examination of the nose. CT scanning is excellent for

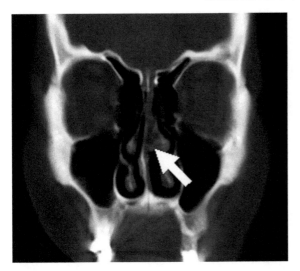

Figure 2.1.9 Coronal CT scan of a 67-year-old female patient with a small defect of the left crista galli and a soft tissue mass extending medially to the left middle turbinate (white arrow). Histology confirmed an esthesioneuroblastoma.

demonstrating opacification, mass effect, or bone destruction. It also allows an evaluation of the orbital apex, infratemporal fossa, posterior ethmoid sinus, cribriform and pterygoid plates, and sphenoid sinus. MRI with gadolinium differentiates an obstructed sinus with fluid collection from a space-occupying lesion. These two modalities complement each other in evaluating and staging tumors of the nasal cavity or the paranasal sinuses. Angiography and PET may be helpful in selected cases. Imaging with an Octreoscan™ (Mallinckrodt Inc, St Louis, USA) is based on the binding of the radiolabeled somatostatin analog, 111In-pentoctreotide (111In-DTPA-D-Pheoctreotide), to a subset of somatostatin receptors in cases of esthesioneuroblastoma.

DIAGNOSIS

Pathologic diagnosis is generally achieved by examining a biopsy from the lesion or the surgical specimen. Imaging is usually required prior to biopsy to avoid serious complications (CSF fistulas in meningoceles or bleeding in highly vascular tumors).

STAGING

The TNM staging system is commonly used for maxillary sinus cancer and nasal cavity and ethmoid sinus cancer (Table 2.1.1). The American Joint Committee on Cancer classification, which is based on Ohngren's original description, emphasizes the size and extent of tumors.

MANAGEMENT

Treatment is either palliative or curative in intent depending on the stage of disease and the patient's overall level of fitness. Most of the tumors of the nasal cavity and paranasal sinuses

Table 2.1.1 TNM Staging System for Maxillary Sinus Cancer and Nasal Cavity and Ethmoid Sinus Cancer

	Maxillary Sinus Cancer
TX	Primary tumor cannot be assessed
T0	No evidence of primary tumor
Tis	Cancer cells are limited to the innermost layer of the mucosa (epithelium). These cancers are known as carcinoma *in situ*
T1	Tumor is only in the tissue lining the sinus (the mucosa) and does not invade bone
T2	Tumor begins to grow into some of the bones of the sinus. (Note: If the cancer grows into the bone of the back part of the sinus, it is classified as T3)
T3	Tumor begins to grow into the bone at the back of the sinus (called the posterior wall) or the tumor has grown into the ethmoid sinus, the tissues under the skin, or the eye socket.
T4a	Tumor grows into other structures such as the skin of the cheek, the eye, the bone at the top of the nose (cribriform plate), the sphenoid sinus, the frontal sinus, or certain parts of the face (the pterygoid plates and the infratemporal fossa).
T4b	Tumor has grown into the area between the nasal cavity and the throat (called the nasopharynx), the brain, the tissue covering the brain (the dura), some parts of the skull (middle cranial fossa, the clivus), or certain nerves.

T Categories for Nasal Cavity and Ethmoid Sinus Cancer

TX	Primary tumor, cannot be assessed
T0	No evidence of primary tumor
Tis	Cancer cells are only in the innermost layer of the mucosa (epithelium). These cancers are known as carcinoma *in situ*
T1	Tumor is only in the nasal cavity or one of the ethmoid sinuses, although it may have grown into the bones of the sinus.
T2	Tumor has grown into other nasal or paranasal cavities
T3	Tumor has grown into the bone of the eye socket, the roof of the mouth (palate), the cribriform plate (the bone that separates the nose from the brain), and/or the maxillary sinus
T4a	Tumor has grown into other structures such as the eye, the skin of the nose, the skin of the cheek, the sphenoid sinus, the frontal sinus, or certain bones in the face (pterygoid plates). Cancers that are T4a are resectable (meaning they can be removed with surgery)
T4b	Tumor is growing into the back of the eye socket, the brain, the dura (the tissue covering the brain), some parts of the skull (the clivus, the middle cranial fossa), certain nerves, or the nasopharynx (the area between the nasal cavity and the throat). Tumors are called T4b when they are not resectable (they cannot be removed with surgery)

N Categories

NX	Nearby (regional) lymph nodes cannot be assessed
N0	Cancer has not spread into the lymph nodes
N1	Cancer has spread to a single lymph node that is on the same side as the tumor and is no larger than 3 cm (slightly larger than an inch)
N2	Cancer has spread to a lymph node that is larger than 3 cm (slightly larger than an inch) but smaller than 6 cm (slightly larger than 2 inches); or cancer has spread to more than one lymph node which are smaller than 6 cm; or cancer is in a lymph node that is not on the same side as the tumor (and the lymph node is smaller than 6 cm).
N3	Cancer has spread to at least one nearby lymph node that is larger than 6 cm (slightly larger than 2 inches)

M Categories

MX	Metastasis cannot be assessed
M0	No distant metastasis
M1	Metastasis present to distant organs such as the lung, brain, or liver.

(Continued)

Table 2.1.1 (Continued)

Stage Groupings			
Stage	T	N	M
Stage 0	Tis	N0	M0
Stage I	T1	N0	M0
Stage II	T2	N0	M0
Stage III	T1 or T2	N1	M0
	T3	N0 or N1	M0
Stage IVA	T1, T2, or T3	N2	M0
	T4a	N0, N1, or N2	M0
Stage IVB	Any T	N3	M0
	T4b	Any N	M0
Stage IVC	Any T	Any N	M1

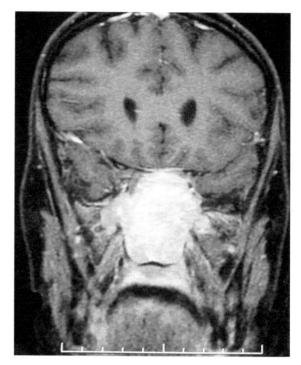

Figure 2.1.11 A coronal MRI scan with gadolinium showing the extensive recurrent squamous cell carcinoma of the nose with dural enhancement (CT presented in Fig. 2.1.10).

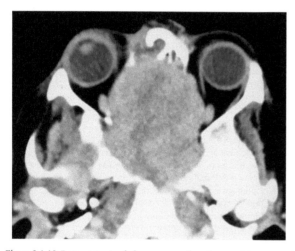

Figure 2.1.10 Recurrent extended squamous cell carcinoma of the nose and paranasal sinuses in a 31-year-old female patient. Postcontrast axial CT scan at the level of orbits. There is an extensive soft tissue mass involving the anterior and posterior ethmoids and destroying the septum and adjacent bony structures. There is extension into both orbits involving the optic nerves.

present with advanced disease, and cure rates are generally poor (Figs. 2.1.10 & 2.1.11). Nodal involvement is infrequent and present in approximately 20% of all cases. Metastases from both nasal cavity and paranasal sinus may occur, but most patients die of direct extension into vital areas of the skull or of rapidly recurring local disease.

Except for T1 mucosal carcinomas, the accepted method of treatment is a combination of radiation therapy and surgery (T2–T4). Destruction of the base of skull (anterior cranial fossa), cavernous sinus, or the pterygoid process; infiltration of the mucous membranes of the nasopharynx; or nonresectable lymph node metastases are relative contraindications to surgery (Fig. 2.1.11). Routine neck dissection or elective neck irradiation is recommended only for patients presenting with positive neck nodes. In resectable tumors, radical surgery is generally performed. This is generally followed by postoperative radiation therapy.

Combined craniofacial approaches may become necessary, including resection of the floor of the anterior cranial fossa. Removal of the eye is performed if the orbit is extensively invaded by cancer. High doses of radiation are necessary to achieve any significant probability of permanent control.

For patients with recurrent disease, chemotherapy should be considered. Chemotherapy for recurrent squamous cell cancer of the head and neck has been shown to be efficacious as palliation and may improve quality of life and length of survival. Various drug combinations including cisplatin, fluorouracil, bleomycin, and methotrexate are known to be effective.

Treatment of tumors of the nasal cavity and paranasal sinuses should be planned on an individual basis because of the complexity involved. Further progress in the treatment of nasal and paranasal sinus cancers could be achieved through better prevention and development of more selective treatments such as endoscopic resection, high-precision radiotherapy, and new chemotherapy drugs. A higher index of suspicion by general practitioners and otolaryngologists may lead to an earlier diagnosis and therefore require less radical treatments with lower morbidity, and quality of life outcomes.

ACKNOWLEDGMENTS

The author is extremely grateful to his new colleagues and the team of the Department of Otolaryngology, Head and Neck Surgery in Bielefeld, Germany.

2.2 Nasopharynx
Holger Sudhoff

ANATOMY

The nasopharynx or nasal part of the pharynx lies posterior to the nasal cavity and superior to the level of the soft palate. Anteriorly it communicates through the choanae with the nasal cavity. The lateral wall contains the pharyngeal ostium of the Eustachian tube. The superior margin merges with the posterior wall and contains abundant lymphoid tissue in pediatric patients known as the adenoids. This tissue usually fades with age but if the adenoids persist into adulthood, it may be confused with a tumor. The nasopharynx does not have many natural barriers to the spread of tumors and has many critical structures immediately adjacent to it. The clivus and the first two vertebral bodies form the posterior bony border of the nasopharynx (Fig. 2.2.1).

Identifiable anatomic structures normally visible on anterior nasal endoscopy include the Eustachian tubes, the cartilaginous ends of the tubes, the torus tubarius and a recessed space, the fossa of Rosenmüller. Occasionally, the endoscopic view is obstructed by crusts, which have to be removed to visualize the underlying pathology.

PRESENTATION

Benign or malignant nasopharyngeal tumors result in few symptoms in the early stages; therefore, most lesions are quite advanced when detected. One should consider normal variants like hyperplastic lymphoid tissue in the nasopharynx when encountering a mass. Benign lesions include juvenile nasopharyngeal angiofibroma (JNA) and neuroma (Fig. 2.2.2A–D). JNA starts adjacent to the sphenopalatine foramen. Large tumors are frequently bi-lobed or dumbbell-shaped, with one portion of the tumor filling the nasopharynx and the other portion extending into the pterygopalatine fossa and occur exclusively in men (Video 6).

Nasopharyngeal carcinoma (Figs. 2.2.3 & 2.2.4) has a lymphoid stroma and is also known as undifferentiated carcinoma of nasopharyngeal type or lymphoepithelioma. Much rarer pathologies include malignant lymphoma, plasmacytoma, adenocarcinoma, melanoma (Figs. 2.2.5, 2.2.6A & B), sarcoma, or chordoma. Once the tumor has expanded from its site of origin in the lateral wall of the nasopharynx, it may obstruct the nasal passages, resulting in a nasal discharge or nosebleed. Obstruction of the auditory tubes may cause chronic ear effusion, otitis media, and patients may experience referred pain to the ear. Metastasis of malignant nasopharyngeal lesions to the lymph nodes of the neck may also be the first noticeable sign of the disease. Tumor invasion into the skull base occurs in approximately 25% of cases and may lead to cranial nerve (CN) palsy. CN V and CN VI are the most commonly involved, followed by CN III and CN IV. Patients with CN involvement present with diplopia and ocular palsies. Unlike malignancies of the oral cavity and oropharynx, malignant nasopharyngeal tumors often metastasize to level V lymph nodes. Bilateral metastases are frequent with rates as high as 50% on initial presentation.

EPIDEMIOLOGY

Juvenile angiofibromas account for 0.05% of all head and neck tumors. A frequency of 1:5,000–1:60,000 has been reported in otolaryngology patients. Onset is most commonly in the second decade ranging from 7 to 19 years. JNA is rare in patients more than 25 years. Malignant nasopharyngeal tumors are rare in Europe, the United States, and most other nations, but have a much higher incidence along the southeast coast of China, including Hong Kong and Macao. An association with the Epstein–Barr virus is observed, but other risk factors have also been found. This is largely due to their diet which involves consumption of salted vegetables, fish, and meat. Current epidemiologic and experimental data suggest at least three major etiologic factors, namely, viral, environmental, and genetic. The age distribution is much younger than for other head and neck cancers. The mean age at diagnosis is 45–55 years, and the annual rates are 23.3 cases per 100,000 men and 8.9 cases per 100,000 women. The male-to-female ratio is approximately 2–3:1. In China, the incidence varies with geography and decreases from southern to northern China, where rates are

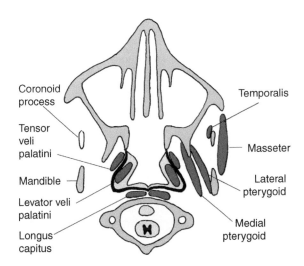

Figure 2.2.1 Schematic illustration of the transverse nasopharyngeal and the suprapalatine region. The heavy black outline indicates the position of the pharyngobasilar fascia. The red-colored areas are muscles.

Coronoid process
Tensor veli palatini
Mandible
Levator veli palatini
Longus capitus
Temporalis
Masseter
Lateral pterygoid
Medial pterygoid

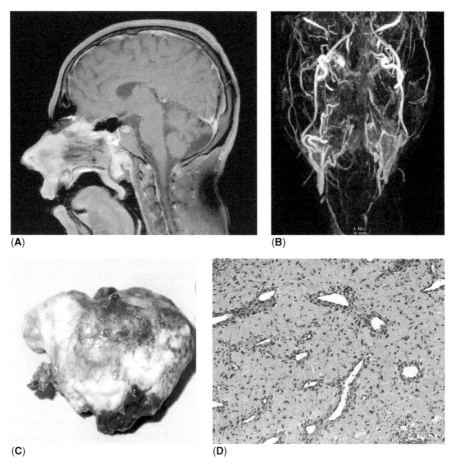

(A)

(B)

(C)

(D)

Figure 2.2.2 (**A**) Juvenile nasopharyngeal angiofibroma (JNA) in a 21-year-old male patient. Lateral MRI view showing a JNR in the postnasal space. An anterior nasal packing became necessary after a biopsy resulting in heavy nose bleeding. (**B**) Angiography shows the branches of the external carotid system to be the primary feeders prior to embolization. (**C**) Surgical specimen after tumor removal via midfacial degloving. (**D**) JNA is usually encapsulated and composed of vascular tissue and fibrous stroma with coarse or fine collagen fibers. Vessels are thin-walled, lack elastic fibers, have absent or incomplete smooth muscle, and vary in appearance from stellate or staghorn to barely conspicuous because of stromal compression. Localized areas of myxomatous degeneration may be observed in the stroma (HE staining).

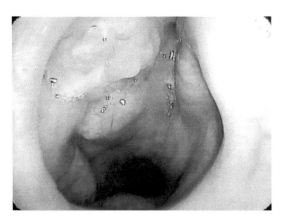

Figure 2.2.3 Endoscopic view from the left nasal cavity of a large nasopharyngeal carcinoma arising from the right side and protruding into the left side of postnasal space, around the back of the septum.

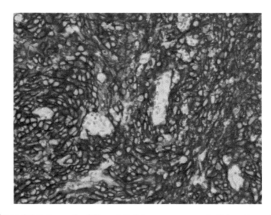

Figure 2.2.4 A poorly differentiated tumor composed of densely packed hyperchromatic cells with a raised nuclear:cytoplasmic ratio. It shows membranous positivity for pan-cytokeratins corroborating a diagnosis of nasopharyngeal carcinoma.

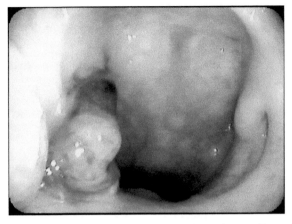

Figure 2.2.5 Metastatic malignant melanoma arising from right Eustachian cushion.

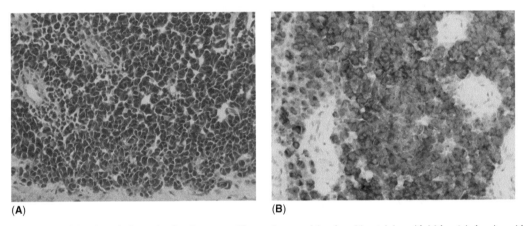

(A) **(B)**

Figure 2.2.6 (A) Sheets of densely packed, angulated melanocytes with prominent nuclei and positive staining with Melan-A in keeping with mucosal melanoma (B).

2–3 cases per 100,000 persons per year. In Europe and America, the risk is increased in first-generation persons of Chinese descent.

IMAGING

Preferred examinations include the following: clinical examination of the neck, rigid or fiberoptic nasal examination, CT scanning of the nasopharynx and neck, and MRI of the nasopharynx and neck. MRI is often more helpful than CT in depicting abnormalities and in defining the extent of tumors (Figs. 2.2.7–2.2.9). Angiography and PET may be helpful in selected cases (Figs. 2.2.2B). Angiography shows the branches of the primary feeders that may be embolized prior to surgery.

Diagnosis

Pathologic diagnosis is generally achieved by examining biopsy specimens from the nasopharyngeal mass of the surgical specimen

(exclude JNA by imaging to avoid potentially life-threatening bleeding from biopsies in an outpatient setting). Epstein–Barr virus serology may be helpful.

STAGING

Different staging systems exist for JNAs. The two most commonly used are those of Sessions and Fisch (Table. 2.2.1). The TNM staging system is commonly used for nasopharyngeal cancer (NPC) (Table. 2.2.2).

MANAGEMENT

Preoperative embolization can be accomplished using reabsorbable microparticulate substances (e.g., Gelfoam® (Pfizer, New York, NY, U.S.A.), polyvinyl alcohol, and dextran microspheres) or nonabsorbable microparticulates. This helps to limit blood loss during surgery for JNAs. With improvement in diagnostic imaging techniques and preoperative embolization,

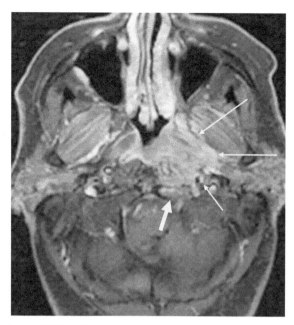

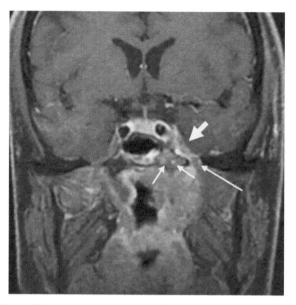

Figure 2.2.7 Nasopharyngeal carcinoma with a skull base invasion. Axial post-gadolinium fatsat T1 images at nasopharyngeal level. Large left nasopharyngeal mass (arrows) extending through pharyngobasilar fascia and infiltrating parapharyngeal fat. Note the encasement of the internal carotid artery (short arrow) and infiltration of the left clivus (thick arrow).

Figure 2.2.9 Coronal fatsat T1 post-gadolinium images at the level of pituitary gland. Nasopharyngeal mass extending laterally into the parapharyngeal and masticator spaces with involvement of the foramen ovale (arrow). Cephalid extension via the foramen lacerum (short white arrows) into the skull base. Note the pathological enhancement of the left cavernous sinus (thick arrow).

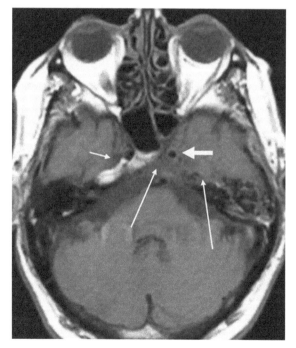

Figure 2.2.8 Axial T1 at the level of Meckel's cave. Encasement and narrowing of the intracavernous internal carotid artery (thick arrow), infiltration of clivus and petrous apex (long arrows), and Meckel's cave. Normal right Meckel's cave (short arrow). Note that the secretions in the left middle ear/mastoid air cells are secondary to Eustachion tube obstruction.

the need for blood transfusion has been greatly reduced. Hormonal therapy or radiotherapy is used in some places but generally surgical resection via different approaches is the gold standard. Approaches are based on the extension and localization of the JNA and comprise the following: intranasal endoscopic surgery; lateral rhinotomy; transpalatal, transmaxillary (e.g., midfacial degloving), or sphenoethmoidal route that is used for small tumors; or the infratemporal fossa, facial translocation or extended anterior subcranial approaches when the tumor has a large lateral extension.

Treatment of nasopharyngeal tumors should be planned on an individual basis because of the complexity involved. It is either palliative or curative in intent depending on the stage of disease and the patient's overall level of fitness in NPC. Because NPC occurs in an anatomical site which is poorly accessible to surgeons, and is often at an advanced stage at presentation, the most effective means of treatment is generally radiation therapy, either with or without concurrent chemotherapy. While the undifferentiated subtype of NPC is highly radiosensitive, this is less true of the more differentiated subtypes. Most of the tumors of the nasopharynx present with advanced disease; so the cure rates are generally poor. Except for T1 mucosal carcinomas, the accepted method of treatment is a combination of radiation therapy and surgery (T2–T4). Destruction of the base of skull (anterior cranial fossa), cavernous sinus, or the pterygoid process; infiltration of the mucous membranes of the nasopharynx; or nonresectable lymph node metastases are relative contraindications to

Table 2.2.1 Tumor Staging Systems for Nasopharyngeal Angiofibroma

Classification according to Sessions	
Stage IA	Tumor limited to posterior nares and/or nasopharyngeal vault
Stage IB	Tumor involving posterior nares and/or nasopharyngeal vault with involvement of at least 1 paranasal sinus
Stage IIA	Minimal lateral extension into pterygomaxillary fossa
Stage IIB	Full occupation of pterygomaxillary fossa with or without superior erosion of orbital bones
Stage IIIA	Erosion of skull base (i.e., middle cranial fossa/pterygoid base); minimal intracranial extension
Stage IIIB	Extensive intracranial extension with or without extension into cavernous sinus
Classification According to Fisch	
Stage I	Tumors limited to nasal cavity, nasopharynx with no bony destruction
Stage II	Tumors invading pterygomaxillary fossa, paranasal sinuses with bony destruction
Stage III	Tumors invading infratemporal fossa, orbit and/or parasellar region remaining lateral to cavernous sinus
Stage IV	Tumors invading cavernous sinus, optic chiasmal region, and/or pituitary fossa

Table 2.2.2 TNM Staging System for Nasopharyngeal Cancer

Primary Tumor (T)	
TX	Primary tumor not assessable
T0	No evidence of primary tumor
Tis	Carcinoma *in situ*
T1	Tumor confined to the nasopharynx
T2	Tumor extending to soft tissues of oropharynx and/or nasal fossa
T2a	Without parapharyngeal extension
T2b	With parapharyngeal extension
T3	Tumor invading bone structures and/or paranasal sinuses
T4	Tumor with intracranial extension and/or involvement of CNs, infratemporal fossa, hypopharynx, or orbit
Regional Lymph Nodes (N)	
NX	Regional lymph nodes not assessable
N0	No regional lymph node metastasis
N1	Unilateral metastasis in lymph node(s), 6 cm or less in greatest dimension, above the supraclavicular fossa
N2	Bilateral metastasis in lymph node(s), 6 cm or less in greatest dimension, above the supraclavicular fossa
N3	Metastasis in a lymph node(s)
N3a	Greater than 6 cm in dimension
N3b	Extension to the supraclavicular fossa
Distant Metastasis (M)	
MX	Distant metastasis not assessable
M0	No distant metastasis
M1	Distant metastasis

(*Continued*)

Table 2.2.2 (*Continued*)

AJCC/UICC Stages			
Stage 0	Tis	N0	M0
Stage I	T1	N0	M0
Stage IIA	T2a	N0	M0
Stage IIB			
	T1	N1	M0
	T2	N1	M0
	T2a	N1	M0
	T2b	N0	M0
	T2b	N1	M0
Stage III			
	T1	N2	M0
	T2a	N2	M0
	T2b	N2	M0
	T3	N0	M0
	T3	N1	M0
	T3	N2	M0
Stage IVA			
	T4	N0	M0
	T4	N1	M0
	T4	N2	M0
Stage IVB	Any T	N3	M0
Stage IVC	Any T	Any N	M1

surgery. Routine neck dissection or elective neck irradiation is recommended only for patients presenting with positive neck nodes. In those tumors that are operable, radical surgery is generally performed. This is commonly followed by postoperative radiation therapy.

Radiation therapy must be carried to high doses for any significant probability of permanent control. For patients with recurrent disease, chemotherapy should be considered. Chemotherapy for recurrent cancer of the head and neck has been shown to be efficacious as palliation and may improve quality of life and length of survival. Various drug combinations including cisplatin, fluorouracil, bleomycin, and methotrexate are effective. Patients with locally advanced disease have poor treatment outcomes after definitive radiotherapy, especially those with cervical lymph nodes who clinically test positive, those with CN involvement, and those with invasion of the skull base. These patients often develop distant metastases despite control of locoregional disease. Most recurrences occur within five years of diagnosis, but late relapses are possible.

ACKNOWLEDGMENTS
The author is extremely grateful to his new colleges and team in the Department of Otolaryngology, Head and Neck Surgery in Bielefeld, Germany.

2.3 Oral cavity
Richard C. W. James

DEFINITION
The oral cavity is limited anteriorly by the vermilion border of the lips, including the labial surfaces, buccal surfaces, the tooth bearing regions of the upper and lower jaws, the hard palate, and the floor of the mouth; it is limited posteriorly by the palatoglossal arch and the junction with the posterior tongue by the circumvallate papillae.

EXAMINATION OF THE ORAL CAVITY
Examination of the oral cavity must be systematic in order to inspect all these areas. It is essential to have good lighting and to use suitable instruments in order to retract tissues adequately.

The floor of the mouth, buccal and lingual sulci, and retromolar areas are best examined using a mouth mirror with a short handle. A gauze square is a useful adjunct as it helps in wiping debri off the mucosal surfaces and may reveal underlying erythema or contact bleeding.

"AT-RISK SITES"
Approximately 75% of oral squamous cell carcinomas (SCCs) are located in the tongue, floor of mouth, and the retromolar trigone. It is suggested that the floor of mouth acts as a "gutter" area and thus carcinogens may gravitate to this area exerting a more pronounced effect on the mucosa.

Second primary SCCs of the upper aero-digestive tract are present in 9% of cases; these are synchronous tumors (arising at the same time) in 30% and metachronous (most common during the first three years of diagnosis) in the remainder.

RISK FACTORS
The consumption of tobacco is recognized as a major risk factor for the development of SCC. Approximately 90% of patients are either current or past smokers.

Alcohol though in itself not a risk factor, acts as a co-carcinogen with tobacco. It is believed that the lipid solubility of alcohol facilitates transportation of carcinogens to the basal layer of oral epithelium.

Betel nut used by south Asian populations is recognized by the International Agency for research on Cancer to be a known carcinogen.

PREMALIGNANT LESIONS
Coexistent white patches are seen in approximately 48% of histologically proven SCCs. Leukoplakia, defined by the World Health Organization as "a white patch or plaque that cannot be characterized clinically or pathologically as any other disease" is recognized as the main potentially malignant oral lesion seen; a malignant transformation rate of 3–33% over 10 years is reported. "Erythroplakia," which has a similar definition but is characterized as a red lesion, though seen less often, has a higher potential to undergo malignant change (Fig. 2.3.1).

"Lichen planus," a mucocutaneous disease that may affect the oral cavity, is recognized as a potentially premalignant condition. There are various presentations; reticular is the most common, usually arising in the buccal mucosa. Classically this has fine white striae against a reddish background and is bilaterally symmetrical. Further presentations include papular, plaque-like, and bullous types. An erosive and an ulcerative type are recognized to have the highest risk of malignant transformation. Lichen planus of any type affecting the tongue is a recognized risk factor in patients who are neither smokers nor excessive drinkers.

"Oral submucous fibrosis," characterized as immobile pale mucosa and associated with the use of betel nut, is a premalignant lesion with a 7% transformation rate. Examining such patients may be difficult owing to associated trismus.

It is advised that all red, white, and mixed lesions present for longer than three weeks should undergo biopsy; malignant transformation of leukoplakias or potentially malignant lesions is not predictable based solely on clinical features.

Patients with premalignant lesions may develop malignant disease. It is important to emphasize smoking and alcohol cessation to patients. Severe dysplasia and *in-situ* carcinoma (Fig. 2.3.2) require excision with margin control; CO_2 laser has been used after histological confirmation for the treatment of moderate dysplasia. Regular follow-up is also required for lichen planus, especially for erosive types and when located in at-risk sites to monitor changes suggestive of malignant transformation.

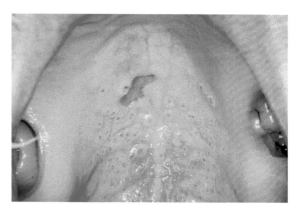

Figure 2.3.1 A smoker's palate showing features of necrotizing sialometaplasia.

ORAL SCC
Presentation
Early SCCs may be asymptomatic, and can be easily missed without careful examination despite the fact that the oral cavity is accessible for thorough evaluation with minimal equipment. The presentation may be classical, as an indurated ulcer with contact bleeding and underlying fixation. Other classical features include erythroplakia, fixation, and either a spontaneously exfoliated tooth (in the absence of generalized periodontal disease) or a dental extraction socket that fails to heal (Figs. 2.3.3–2.3.7).

As oral lesions may be asymptomatic, the initial presentation may be an enlarged, metastatic lymph node corresponding to the area of lymphatic drainage—level I (submandibular) for floor-of-the-mouth SCC and level II/III for anterior tongue SCC.

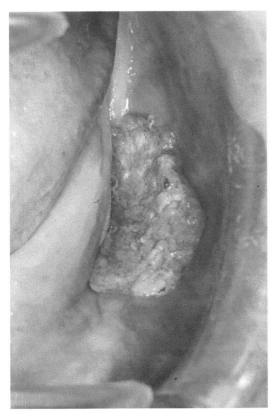

Figure 2.3.2 Severe dysplasia and carcinoma *in situ* left mandibular alveolus.

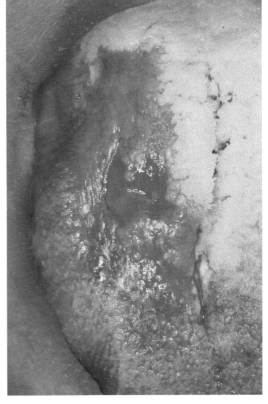

Figure 2.3.4 Squamous cell carcinoma, dorsum of right side of tongue.

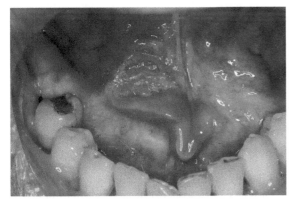

Figure 2.3.3 Floor-of-the-mouth squamous cell carcinoma.

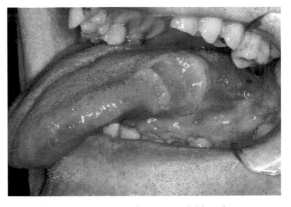

Figure 2.3.5 Squamous cell carcinoma, left lateral tongue.

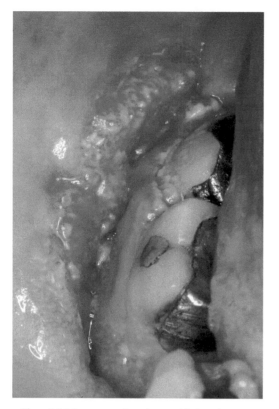

Figure 2.3.6 Squamous cell carcinoma, right buccal mucosa.

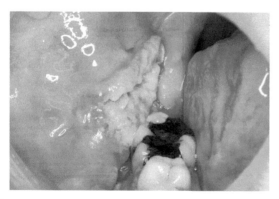

Figure 2.3.7 Squamous cell carcinoma, right buccal and retromolar mucosa.

Epidemiology

SCCs account for approximately 90% of all intraoral malignancies. Approximately 24,000 new cases are diagnosed annually in the United States with around 8000 annual deaths attributed to this disease. This accounts for 14–24% of all head and neck malignancies. The reported highest incidence is in India, where it accounts for 20–30% of all malignancies. Within the United Kingdom the incidence varies from 8 per 100,000 in the Thames and Oxford regions to 13–15 per 100,000 in Wales. There were 2329 new cases of mouth, lip, and oral cavity malignancies and 782 deaths recorded in England for the year 2000.

The age at presentation is generally above 40 years, though cases are seen in a significantly younger age group. The youngest reported case was a SCC affecting the hard palate in a 6-year old. The male to female ratio is 2:1.

Almost half of new cases present with regional lymph node involvement often associated with social and economic deprivation.

It is estimated that 90% of patients are tobacco and alcohol consumers. The risks associated with heavy tobacco use are increased by six times, but where the alcohol intake is greater than 30 units per week, the combined effect is an increase of 24–80 times that of abstainers. Human papilloma viruses (HPV), in particular HPV16 and 18 have been shown to be associated with SCC. These may be a factor in the development of 20–30% of malignancies, in particular those patients who are nonsmokers and occasional drinkers.

Staging

Oral SCCs are staged according to the International Union Against Cancer (UICC) TNM system sixth edition 2002.

Tx: Tumor cannot be assessed

T0: No evidence of primary tumor

Tis: Carcinoma *in situ*

T1: Tumor up to 2 cm in maximum dimension

T2: Tumor between 2 cm and 4 cm in maximum dimension

T3: Tumor greater than 4 cm in greatest dimension

T4a: Tumor invasion of cortical bone, into deep/extrinsic muscle of tongue (genioglossus, hyoglossus, palatoglossus, and styloglossus), maxillary sinus or skin of face

T4b: Tumor invades masticator space, pterygoid plates, or skull base or encases internal carotid artery

Note that superficial erosion alone of tooth/tooth socket by gingival primary is not sufficient to classify a tumor as T4.

Investigations

The clinical examination may need to be supplemented with an examination and biopsy under general anesthesia. This may be useful in order to delineate the extent of the primary and may reveal a second primary tumor. More commonly, a diagnostic biopsy is performed under local anesthesia. There may be justification in obtaining imaging prior to biopsy where the diagnosis is clinically obvious, as distortion of the primary tumor on imaging may result.

The panoramic dental radiograph, though not a sensitive investigation, is performed in order to assess gross bone involvement. It is extremely useful as it provides information concerning the dental status of the patient; in particular where radiotherapy forms part of the patient's treatment there is a risk of osteoradionecrosis should dental extractions be required subsequently (Figs. 2.3.8 & 2.3.9).

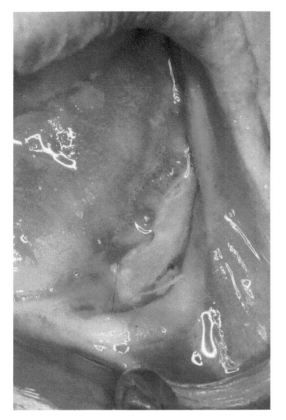

Figure 2.3.8 Osteoradionecrosis of the left mandible.

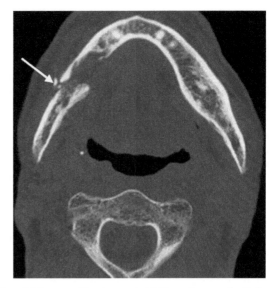

Figure 2.3.9 54 year old male treated with Chemotherapy and radiotherapy for T4 N2c squamous cell carcinoma tonsil 4 yrs ago. Right jaw discomfort. Postradiotherapy osteoradionecrosis. Axial CT images of the mandible on bone settings. Loss of normal trabecular pattern in the body of the right mandible together with frank bone destruction and a pathological fracture (arrow).

Chest radiography is performed to assess distant spread of the disease. This may be substituted by chest CT where a patient is deemed to be at high risk of either a lung primary or metastasis.

The use of magnetic resonance (MRI) is generally preferable to CT in order to assess the primary tumor, the degree of involvement of adjacent tissue, and regional lymphatics. However, this is a highly sensitive investigation and may reveal false positives in so far as bone involvement is concerned. For this reason CT may be useful in addition to further evaluate, for example, the orbital floor and the mandible. MRI also has a false-positive rate in detecting lymph node involvement and approximately 30% of patients will have occult metastases. Therefore, imaging cannot be relied upon to determine regional lymphatic involvement.

Management

Management of the primary tumor will usually involve surgical excision with an adequate margin (1 cm) of normal tissue. A degree of tissue shrinkage, particularly with tongue and buccal mucosa of the order of 20% may reduce the reported histological margins. Floor-of-the-mouth tumors and tumors that involve alveolar mucosa may have invaded the adjacent mandible. In this situation either a rim resection or segmental resection

may be required. Elevating the periosteum and subsequent examination of both periosteum and the underlying bone will give valuable information as to the degree of involvement. A rim resection is performed if no involvement is apparent. Where definite invasion is seen, a segmental resection is performed. This is because of an intramedullary spread and a poor radio sensitivity of the involved bone.

Accessing the primary site for confident resection may require a mandibulotomy. This is particularly useful for lateral and more posterior tongue tumors, but may also be useful in gaining access to the posterior floor of mouth and retromolar areas. Where tumors have extended into regional lymphatics in continuity resection may only be possible by mandibulotomy. A paramedian mandibulotomy with a lip splitting approach gives excellent access. With a good approximation of the lips, esthetics is generally very good. Performing the bone cuts anterior to the mental foramen and between mandibular teeth roots is important to prevent iatrogenic damage to adjacent tissues. A mandibular lingual releasing operation often referred to as "the visor drop down" approach provides an excellent access to the whole tongue and floor of mouth into the neck. It is important to ensure accurate reattachment of genioglossus and geniohyoid to the genial tubercle with this approach during wound closure. Significant effects on speech, swallowing, and chewing may otherwise result.

Cervical lymphatics are involved in approximately 50% of patients at presentation. These may be occult. A neck dissection is required (radical and modified radical) where disease is present; a staging neck dissection of affected levels (I–IV) is required where a risk of occult nodes is greater than 20%. A high risk for metastasis is recognized with T1/T2 tongue SCC where thickness is greater than 4 mm.

Small defects can be managed with primary closure. The tongue may be sutured anteriorly to posterior—subsequent adaptation will allow good function. Skin grafts can be used in floor-of-the-mouth defects, though scarring will result, reducing tongue mobility and thus potentially reducing function. Local flaps such as nasolabial flaps may be used for small anterior defects.

Larger defects of the tongue, floor of the mouth, and buccal tissues require free tissue (microvascular) reconstruction. Where soft tissue defects only are present, a radial forearm flap or anterolateral thigh flap is most often used. Where mandibular defects require reconstruction, a free-fibular reconstruction is commonly used. Other methods of composite reconstruction include vascularized iliac crest (based on the deep circumflex artery) and the scapula (based on the circumflex scapular artery). Composite reconstruction allows placement of osseointegrated implants. This will provide good functional outcome, improve appearance, and maintain good quality of life.

Maxillary defects traditionally have been managed with prosthetic obturation. These devices are reasonably well tolerated and allow regular inspection of the primary site. With the possibility of osseointegrated implants, composite reconstruction is increasingly carried out using vascularized iliac crest, scapular and free fibular grafts. Implantation can be carried out at the time of graft placement or subsequently

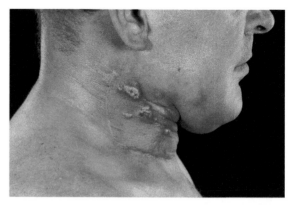

Figure 2.3.10 Cutaneous metastases, right neck following neck dissection.

following a detailed study of the resulting reconstruction (Fig. 2.3.10).

Five-Year Survival and Stage at Presentation
The overall five-year survival of SCC of the tongue is 42% and oral cavity is 47%. When analyzed into stages, the two-year survival is as follows:

Stage I: Early disease, 87.5%
Stage II: Locally advanced disease, 68.6%
Stage III: Lymph node involved, 52.5%
Stage IV: Metastatic disease, 46%

2.4.1 Oropharynx tumors
Tom Wilson

The oropharynx is a part of the pharynx and located as the conduit between the oral cavity, nasopharynx, and hypopharynx. The margins are the anterior faucial pillars, the tongue posterior to the circumvallate papillae (tongue base), the valleculae, the inferior mucosal surface of the soft palate and the posterior pharyngeal wall mucosa.

PRESENTATION
The majority of tumors are squamous cell carcinomas (SCCs; 90%) followed by non-Hodgkin's lymphoma and rarely minor salivary gland carcinomas or other soft tissue sarcomas. Tumors most commonly are found in the tonsils or tonsillar fossa, either visualized directly as a craggy enlarged tonsil or felt as a painful ulcerated lesion (chap. 2.4.2). Occasionally, they may involve the glossopharyngeal nerve with pain radiating to the ipsilateral ear. Tumors involving the pterygoid muscles will present with trismus (an inability to open the mouth fully). Tumors can also arise in the tongue base where they often present late or even silently as a coincidental mass while investigating the primary source of a metastatic neck node (lateral neck mass).

Non Hodgkin's lymphomas will present as unilaterally enlarged painless tonsillar or tongue base mass with or without constitutional upset (B symptoms) (see clinical photo, chap. 2.4.3).

Minor salivary gland carcinomas classically present on the inferior surface of the soft palate or lateral pharyngeal wall as firm nodular lesions and are likely to be mucoepidermoid carcinomas or adenoid cystic carcinomas.

EPIDEMIOLOGY
The commonest tumor of the oropharynx is SCC. Incidence in the United States is 1.8/100,000 per year with mortality rates being 0.4/100,000 per year. The male to female ratio is 3.5:1 with the commonest presentation being a male over the age of 50. The associated risk factors are chronic tobacco use, betel nut chewing, mate tea drinking, and excessive alcohol consumption. There is also an association with Plummer–Vinson syndrome and human papillomavirus -16 virus infection.

The abundance of lymphatic tissue in the tongue base and tonsils accounts for the oropharynx being the commonest extra nodal site for non-Hodgkin's lymphoma to present in the pediatric population.

CLINICAL APPEARANCE
The oropharynx is assessed by direct vision through the mouth, palpation via the mouth, and a pharyngoscopy either via a fiberoptic nasendoscope in clinic or pharyngoscope under general anesthetic (Figs. 2.4.1.1 & 2.4.1.2).

Leukoplakia is a white patch or plaque-like lesion and erythroleukoplakia appears as a red nonspecific patch. These are both premalignant lesions. SCC appears as an ulcerated exophytic lesion, usually on the tonsil or in the tonsillar fossa (chap. 2.4.2). Tongue base SCC appears as an irregular lesion/ulcer in the tongue base or may be symptomless and not apparent until a pharyngoscopy is undertaken to search for an occult primary site for a lymph node metastases in the neck (Figs. 2.4.1.3 & 2.4.1.4).

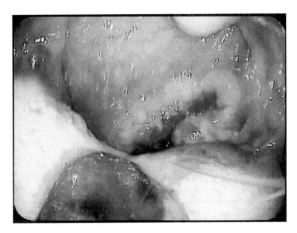

Figure 2.4.1.1 A left lateral pharyngeal wall SCC arising from behind the left tonsil and spreading inferiorly. Viewed through the mouth with a metal tongue depressor inferiorly.

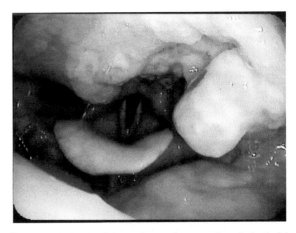

Figure 2.4.1.2 The same lesion as the one above, seen from the level of the soft palate. The lesion is spreading inferiorly to involve the posterior pharyngeal wall.

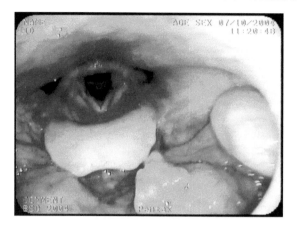

Figure 2.4.1.3 A left tongue base lesion seen from the level of the soft palate.

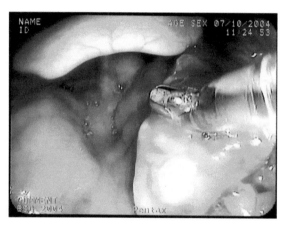

Figure 2.4.1.4 The same lesion as the one above being biopsied under local anesthetic.

Minor salivary gland carcinomas appear as either painless rubbery, occasionally ulcerated, swellings which can appear fluctuant and represent mucoepidermoid carcinoma or else appear as a larger slowly growing, painful mass representing an adenoid cystic carcinoma with its tendency for perineural infiltration.

IMAGING

SCC of the oropharynx, especially of the tongue base, has an increased tendency for late presentation with occult/bilateral nodal metastases and synchronous aero-digestive tract malignancy. It is important to image patients with this in mind so imaging of the neck and chest with MRI and/or CT allowing staging of the disease prior to treatment planning is mandatory (Figs. 2.4.1.5 & 2.4.1.6).

Non-Hodgkin's lymphoma presenting as an oropharyngeal mass will also need imaging to allow disease staging prior to treatment planning via imaging of the neck, chest, abdomen, and pelvis with MRI and/or CT (chaps 2.4.2 & 2.4.3).

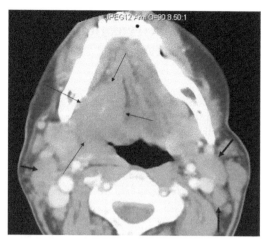

Figure 2.4.1.5 An axial postcontrast CT through base of tongue and tonsillar fossae. A large mass at the right base of the tongue extending into floor of mouth and tonsillar fossa. Bilateral level 2 lymphadenopathy. Arrows = mass. Thick arrows = level 2 lymphadenopathy.

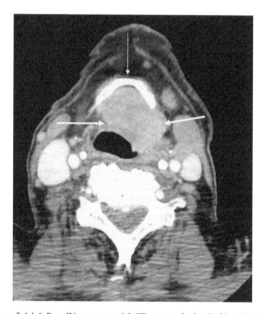

Figure 2.4.1.6 Post-IV contrast axial CT scan at the level of hyoid. A large mass occupying pre-epiglottic space extending into valleculae. Arrow = hyoid bone. Thick arrows = mass.

STAGING

T1: Tumor <2 cm

T2: Tumor >2 cm to 4 cm

T3: Tumor >4 cm

T4a: Tumor extends to larynx, deep/extrinsic muscle of tongue, medial pterygoid, hard palate, and mandible.

T4b: Tumor extends to lateral pterygoid muscle, pterygoid plate, lateral nasopharynx, skull base, and carotid artery.

MANAGEMENT

Management of SCC of the oropharynx will depend upon the disease stage and the exact site of the primary tumor. Early stage disease (T1 or T2 with no clinical evidence of neck metastases) will be treated either by primary surgery or external beam radiotherapy with treatment of the ipsilateral neck by either a neck dissection or radiotherapy and treatment of the contralateral neck as well if the primary lesion is known to be in the tongue base or near the midline. Advanced stage disease (III or IV) can also be treated by either surgery or radiotherapy depending on the exact site of the primary tumor. Surgical resection of the disease is compromised by the need to obtain clear surgical margins and resulting functional compromise on resecting significant parts of the oropharynx. Surgical resection will be supplemented with reconstruction as necessary. If the neck and primary site are treated by primary surgery then the patient will be recommended for postoperative radiotherapy with concomitant chemotherapy (cisplatin).

Non Hodgkin's lymphoma will be treated by the hematological oncologists using chemotherapy.

Minor salivary gland carcinomas will be treated by surgery and postoperative radiotherapy.

2.4.2 Tonsil tumors
Hemi Patel

PRESENTATION

Tonsillar tumors may present in a variety of ways. There location in a relatively large oropharynx and the deep invaginations of its structure make late presentation with advanced disease much more likely than other head and neck sites. Sore throat, ipsilateral otalgia, globus or lump sensation, and bleeding are all possible presenting symptoms. However, patients present most commonly with an exophytic tonsillar mass or an isolated lump in the neck.

Trismus is ominous as it suggests involvement of the parapharyngeal space.

Lymphatic spread is common, affecting 50% of patients at presentation. The most common nodes affected are the ipsilateral jugulodigastric and upper deep cervical nodes.

EPIDEMIOLOGY

Tonsillar tissue is rich in lymphatics, blood vessels, nerve fibers, and epithelium. Malignant tumors can arise from them all. Squamous cell carcinoma (SCC) and lymphoma account for more than 95%.

Squamous Cell Carcinomas

SCC of the oropharynx is uncommon. It represents 10–15% of all head and neck cancers and accounts for 0.3–0.5% of all registered malignancies. The incidence in the United Kingdom is approximately 6–8 per million, they are four times more common in men and develop in the fifth decade of life or later. They have a peak incidence in the 6th–7th decades.

In the oropharynx, the tonsil is the most common subsite (50%) involved, followed by the tongue base (35%), soft palate (10%), and the posterior pharyngeal wall (5%). SCC makes up over 70% of malignant tonsillar tumors.

Currently accepted risk factors for SCC include smoking and alcohol abuse, gastroesophageal reflux disease, a diet deficient in fruits and vegetables, and chewing of betel quid. Infection with human papilloma virus (HPV) has also been implicated.

Lymphoma

These account for 25% of malignant tonsillar tumors. They are usually diagnosed in the 6th or 7th decade of life, but can also occur in the very young; hence the reason for considering tonsillectomy in unilateral enlargement of the tonsils in children.

HISTOPATHOLOGY AND CLINICAL APPEARANCE

A core biopsy and tonsillectomy are ways of obtaining diagnostic tissue. SCCs in this area are usually moderately to poorly differentiated, although undifferentiated and nonkeratinizing variants occur with some regularity.

Most tonsillar lymphomas are diffuse non-Hodgkin's large B cell, but accurate type determination is crucial (see clinical photo, chap. 2.4.3).

Macroscopically, tonsillar tumors can vary from a slight enlargement or firmness of the tonsil to an exophytic fungating mass with central ulceration. (Figs. 2.4.2.1–2.4.2.3).

IMAGING

Accurate staging can only be achieved with imaging.

PET scanning is useful when trying to locate an unknown primary tumor which has spread to cervical lymph nodes. The scan should be carried out prior to any biopsies as these areas of

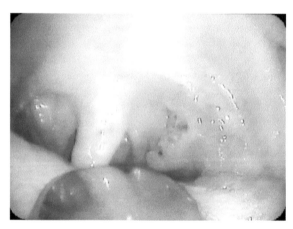

Figure 2.4.2.1 Left tonsillar carcinoma viewed from the mouth.

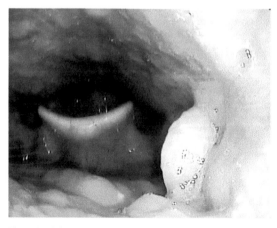

Figure 2.4.2.2 Left tonsillar tumor viewed from the postnasal space.

"trauma" will give false-positive results. In Figure 2.4.2.4, the tonsils are both "hot," and a bilateral synchronous SCC was uncovered.

CT scanning of the neck is vital in assessing the extent of the primary tumor and nodal metastasis to the neck.

MRI is superior in assessing the tumor size and soft tissue invasion in tumors of the oropharynx (tonsil and base of tongue) and should be performed where available Figs. 2.4.2.5 & 2.4.2.6.

A chest radiograph and CT should be performed to assess the presence of any lung metastasis.

T-STAGING SYSTEM (SPECIFIC FOR OROPHARYNX)

T1: Tumor ≤2 cm

T2: Tumor >2 cm–4 cm

T3: Tumor >4 cm

T4a: Bone, muscle, sinus, skin involvement

T4b: Masticator space, pterygoid plates, skull base, internal carotid artery

STAGE GROUPINGS

Stage I	T1	
Stage II	T2	
Stage III	T1, T2	N1
	T3	N0, N
Stage IVa	T1, T2, T3	N2
	T4a	N0, N1, N2
Stage IVb	T4b	Any N
Stage IVc	Any T	Any N
	M1	

MANAGEMENT

If the diagnosis of a lymphoma is made, the patient should be referred to an appropriate hematologist for specialist treatment.

The treatment of tonsillar SCC is complex and should be individualized to the patient. The extent of treatment and the modality depends on the stage of the disease, the fitness of the patients, and their wishes after appropriate counseling and local expertise.

Early Cancer (Stage I and II)

Primary resection, with appropriate reconstruction and selective neck dissection (levels II–IV), and external beam radiotherapy encompassing both primary tumor and neck levels II–IV are viable options with similar outcomes.

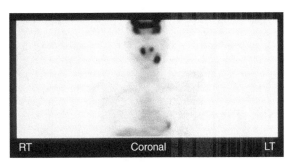

Figure 2.4.2.4 A PET scan showing an uptake in the "branchial cyst" and an asymmetrical uptake in the tonsils.   *Source*: Price T, Pickles J. Bilateral synchronous tonsillar carcinomas: The role of FDG-PET scanning in the search for the occult primary tumour. Journal of Laryngology & Otology 2006; 120 4: 334–337.

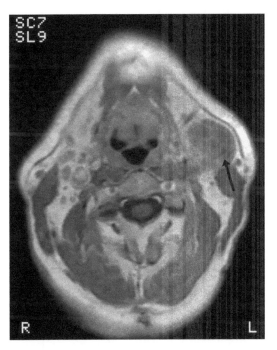

Figure 2.4.2.5 An MRI showing a loculated lesion consistent with a metastatic level 2/3 lymph node (black arrow).   *Source*: Same as that of Figure 2.4.2.4.

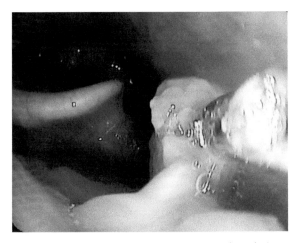

Figure 2.4.2.3 Biopsy of the above lesion under local anesthetic.

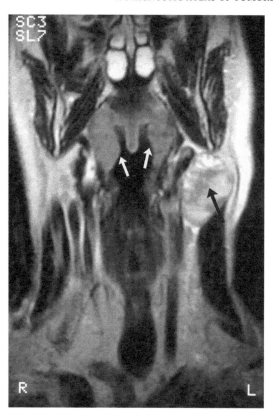

Figure 2.4.2.6 A T2-weighted MRI showing a slightly higher signal in both tonsils (white arrows) than "normal." The metastatic node is indicated by the black arrow. *Source*: Same as that of Figure 2.4.2.4.

Locally Advanced Cancer (Stage III and IV)
Patients may be treated with primary surgery if clear margins can be obtained, or an organ preservation approach with radiotherapy and concurrent chemotherapy.

OUTCOME AND PROGNOSIS
Five-year survival rates of treated tonsillar SCC can be summarized as follows:

Stage I: 80%
Stage II: 70%
Stage III: 40%
Stage IV: 30%

The risk of locoregional recurrence and the propensity to develop a second primary tumor (30%) in these patients make a close follow-up after treatment essential.

2.4.3 Base of tongue tumors
Tim Price

PRESENTATION

Tumors of the base of tongue may be very difficult to diagnose early because of vague symptoms. Therefore, up to three-quarters of patients present with stage III or IV disease. They may present with a sore throat, a foreign body in the throat sensation (globus), referred otalgia, odynophagia (painful swallowing), and altered or muffled speech. Advanced ulcerated tumors may have severe pain and halitosis (an anaerobic smell) because of secondary infection. However, up to 20% of patients will present with a lymph node in the neck and no obvious primary tumor, the so-called occult primary tumor.

These tumors have a poor prognosis because of the high incidence of nodal metastases at presentation (70–85% for T1–T4 tumors). Approximately one-third of patients will have bilateral metastases.

EPIDEMIOLOGY

The male to female ratio is 2.5:1 with the peak incidence in male patients in the 7th decade and in the 6th decade in females. Etiological factors in genetically predisposed individuals include tobacco smoking, with a synergistic effect of alcohol, especially spirits.

HISTOLOGY AND CLINICAL APPEARANCE

The majority of the tumors are squamous cell carcinomas (70%) and lymphomas (25%) with the rest being made up of minor salivary gland tumors. Squamous cell carcinomas tend to be ulcerated, while lymphomas tend to be more bulky and fleshy (Fig. 2.4.3.1A & B) but both can appear exophytic in nature (Figs. 2.4.3.2 & 2.4.3.3). Patients with lymphomas tend to be younger than those with an SCC and may have weight loss and night sweats (B symptoms). It is important to examine the whole of the upper aero-digestive tract as 30% of SCC patients will have a synchronous second primary or will develop a metachronous second primary within 10 years of presentation (Fig. 2.4.3.4).

IMAGING

The best mode of imaging the base of tongue to assess extension into surrounding tissues and lymph nodes in the neck is an MRI scan (Figs. 2.4.3.5 & 2.4.3.6). A chest x-ray or CT chest should be performed.

If biopsies prove a lesion is a lymphoma, the patient should be referred to a lymphoma specialist for further investigation and treatment which usually involves treatment of localized disease with radiotherapy and chemotherapy for systemic disease.

STAGING

The TNM staging system is commonly used.

T1: Tumor 2 cm or less in diameter

T2: Tumor more than 2 cm but not more than 4 cm in greatest dimension

T3: Tumor more than 4 cm in greatest dimension

T4a: Tumor invades the larynx, deep/intrinsic muscle of the tongue, medial pterygoid, hard palate, or mandible.

T4b: Tumor invades lateral pterygoid muscle, pterygoid plates, lateral nasopharynx, or skull base, or encases the carotid artery.

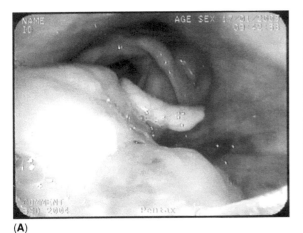

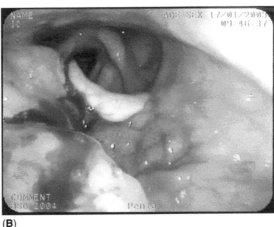

(A)   **(B)**

Figure 2.4.3.1 (**A**) Clinical photograph of large B cell lymphoma of the tongue base and right tonsil. (**B**) Post biopsy.

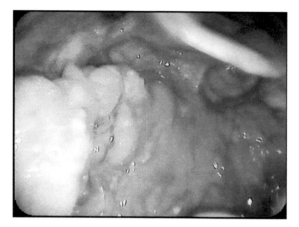

Figure 2.4.3.2 Exophytic right tongue base SCC.

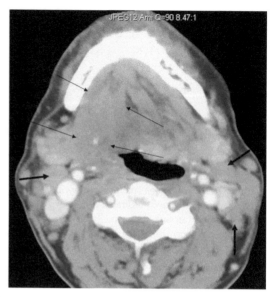

Figure 2.4.3.5 Axial postcontrast CT through the base of the tongue and tonsillar fossae. A large mass in the right base of tongue extending into the floor of the mouth and tonsillar fossa. Bilateral level 2 lymphadenopathy.

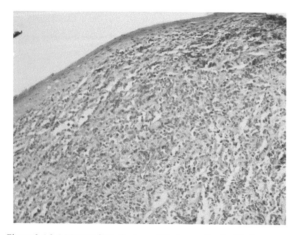

Figure 2.4.3.3 Same lesion as the one above being biopsied under local anesthetic.

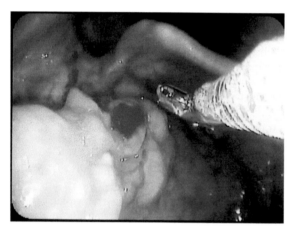

Figure 2.4.3.4 Mucosa from the base of the tongue lined with almost atrophic but nondysplastic squamous cell epithelium. Underneath, there is a diffuse infiltrate of atypical, rather large lymphocytes with features in keeping with a diffuse large B-cell lymphoma (H&E, x200).

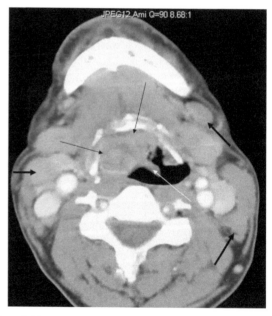

Figure 2.4.3.6 Postcontrast axial CT level of hyoid. Base of the tongue tumor extending into the right vallecula. Enlarged level 2/3 lymph nodes on the right. A mildly enlarged left submandibular lymph node. Arrows = tumor involving the right vallecula. Thick arrows = lymphadenopathy. White arrow = epiglottis.

MANAGEMENT

In the treatment of SCCs the results of radiotherapy and surgery are equivocal, but radiotherapy with or without chemotherapy is favoured because of the better functional outcomes. Brachytherapy with implants is also employed for these tumors. Treatment includes the neck because of the high incidence of nodal involvement and this should include a bilateral neck dissection in those patients with clinically involved neck nodes.

Early lesions can be approached transorally via a paramedian mandibulotomy, and the midline tongue split and the defect reconstructed with myocutaneous free flaps to achieve a good functional result.

Transoral laser surgery is gaining in popularity across the world and tumors are excised using the laser until frozen sections provide a clear margin of excision. The site of the tumor is then left to heal by secondary intention. The postoperative morbidity is less for this type of surgery and patients therefore spend a far shorter time in hospital recovering from the surgery.

Advanced lesions usually require a total glossolaryngectomy in order to get sufficient oncological clearance. This is clearly a very debilitating operation and not frequently performed because of this and the general fitness of the patients. Alternative treatments include induction chemotherapy with radiotherapy preserve the larynx and maintain normal swallowing function.

FIVE-YEAR SURVIVAL RATES

These vary from institution to institution.

Stage I: 50–100%
Stage II: 77–44%
Stage III: 76–45%
Stage IV: 59–11%

2.5.1 Supraglottic tumors
Mike Thomas

PRESENTATION

The most common symptoms for supraglottic tumors include hoarseness, dysphagia, odynophagia, and a neck swelling. Presentation is usually late and as nodal disease is more common, patients are more likely to present with a neck mass. Other symptoms include hemoptysis, dyspnea with stridor, chronic cough, and referred otalgia. Supraglottic cancers tend not to cause noticeable symptoms early in the disease course. Spread of supraglottic tumors often involves structures outside the larynx such as the tongue base, vallecula, piriform fossa and postcricoid region. Persistent sore throat and referred otalgia may indicate tongue base involvement. Inferior spread to the vocal folds and subglottis can occur but it is uncommon. The lymphatic vascularity is denser in the supraglottis accounting for a higher incidence of nodal metastases. Up to 70% of patients can have advanced disease at presentation and the incidence of occult cervical lymph-node metastases is linked to T stage and can range from 20% in T1/T2 tumors to 50% in T3/T4 tumors. The primary echelons of nodal drainage of supraglottic tumors are of levels II, III and IV.

EPIDEMIOLOGY

Supraglottic tumors account for between 27% and 31% of all laryngeal cancers in the United Kingdom and United States of America. In France, Spain, and India the incidence is higher, between 60% and 70%, probably due to different carcinogens. It is commoner in men, usually presenting in the 6th or 7th decades. The mucosa of the supraglottis is composed of nonkeratinizing, stratified squamous epithelium, which changes into a ciliated, pseudostratified, columnar epithelium at the false vocal folds and ventricle. The vast majority of tumors are squamous cell in origin; nonsquamous tumors arise from salivary gland tissue and neuroendocrine cells. Atypical carcinoid is the most frequent neuroendocrine tumor, with 90% of them occurring in the supraglottis; small cell tumors ("oat-cell" carcinomas) are rare but aggressive and often have widespread metastases. Adenoid cystic carcinomas have been described, as have melanomas, lymphomas and Kaposi's sarcomas. There is a 4% incidence of synchronous lesions.

CLINICAL APPEARANCE

The clinical appearance varies from a localized swelling or ulceration affecting one of the four subdivisions of the supraglottic larynx in early stage disease to a large fungating lesion causing significant anatomical distortion, airway compromise, and invasion into adjacent structures. Partial or complete fixation of one or both vocal folds can occur usually in advanced disease. An accurate assessment of the neck is required to assess for cervical node involvement but this may be underestimated clinically. Clinical examination should include palpation of the tongue base. Endoscopic assessment is required together with adequate biopsies Figs. 2.5.1.1–2.5.1.6.

IMAGING

A chest radiograph should be undertaken to exclude a lung primary or metastases; if metastases are shown or if suspicion is high, then a CT scan of the chest is warranted. Imaging studies help to define the spread of the disease into the pre-epiglottic

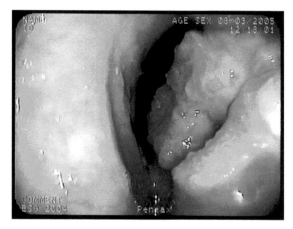

Figure 2.5.1.1 A large supraglottic squamous cell carcinoma spreading inferiorly to involve the left vocal cord.

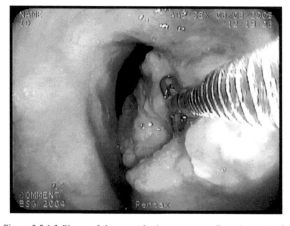

Figure 2.5.1.2 Biopsy of the supraglottic squamous cell carcinoma in the clinic.

and paraglottic spaces together with thyroid cartilage invasion or extralaryngeal submucosal extension. Often, both CT and MRI scanning are needed to accurately assess a supraglottic tumor. Scans also help assess tongue base involvement and spread into cervical nodes. CT and MRI scans can measure the lymph node size; both can show areas of central lucency which suggests tumor involvement. Positron emission tomography scans may help diagnose lesions earlier and more accurately assess recurrence. Both clinical and radiological findings allow accurate staging of the lesion using the TNM staging system Figs. 2.5.1.5, 2.5.1.7, 2.5.1.8.

STAGING

TX: Primary tumor cannot be assessed.

T0: No evidence of primary tumor.

T1: Tumor limited to one subsite of supraglottis with normal vocal cord mobility

T2: Tumor invades the mucosa of more than one adjacent subsite of supraglottis or glottis or region outside the supraglottis (e.g., mucosa of the base of the tongue, vallecula, and medial wall of piriform sinus) without fixation of the larynx

T3: Tumor limited to larynx with vocal cord fixation and/or invades any of the following: postcricoid area, pre-epiglottic tissues, paraglottic space, and/or with minor thyroid cartilage erosion (e.g., inner cortex)

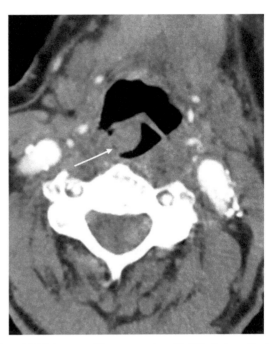

Figure 2.5.1.5 A 73 year old man presenting with difficulty in swallowing. Mediastinal leiomyosarcoma with epiglottic metastasis. Axial postconstrast CT scan, at the level of the supraglottic larynx. A soft tissue mass arising from the right epiglottis.

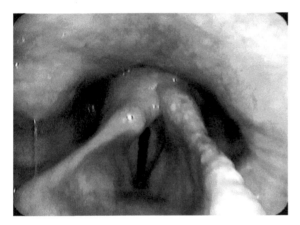

Figure 2.5.1.3 Supraglottic squamous cell carcinoma of the left aryepiglottic fold.

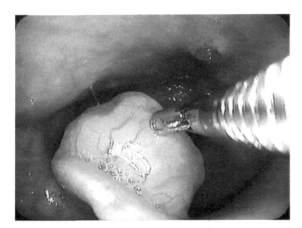

Figure 2.5.1.4 Metastatic leiomyosarcoma of the posterior surface of epiglottis being biopsied in clinic.

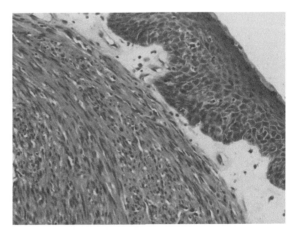

Figure 2.5.1.6 A circumscribed nodule, lying beneath the squamous epithelium, composed of fascicles of moderately pleomorphic spindle cells. The features are those of metastatic leiomyosarcoma.

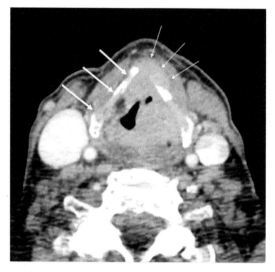

Figure 2.5.1.7 Axial postcontrast CT scan just above false cord level. Pre- and paraglottic fat infiltration anteriorly crossing the midline and on the left. Extralaryngeal spread extending through thyroid cartilage anteriorly (*arrows*). Thick arrows = thyroid cartilage.

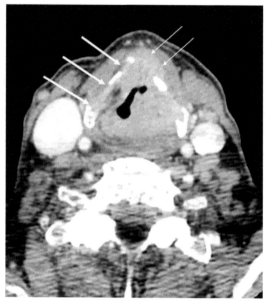

Figure 2.5.1.8 Postcontrast axial CT scan at level of false cord. Pre- and paraglottic fat infiltration anteriorly crossing the midline and on the left. Extralaryngeal spread extending through thyroid cartilage anteriorly (*arrows*). Thick arrows = thyroid cartilage.

T4a: Tumor invades through the thyroid cartilage and/or invades tissues beyond the larynx, e.g., trachea, soft tissues of neck including deep/extrinsic muscle of tongue (genioglossus, hyoglossus, palatoglossus, and styloglossus), strap muscles, thyroid, and esophagus

T4b: Tumor invades prevertebral space or mediastinal structures, or encases the carotid artery.

MANAGEMENT

An appropriate treatment protocol should be selected for each patient, given the anatomic problem, performance status, and clinical expertise of the treatment team involved.

T1: External-beam radiation therapy alone or supraglottic laryngectomy. Endoscopic resection in selected patients.

T2: External-beam radiation therapy alone for small lesions or endoscopic resection in selected patients. Supraglottic laryngectomy or total laryngectomy depending on the location of the tumor. Postoperative radiotherapy for positive or close surgical margins.

T3: Surgery with or without postoperative radiotherapy or definitive radiation therapy with surgery for salvage of radiation failures. Concomitant chemotherapy and radiation therapy, with laryngectomy in patients who show a poor response to chemotherapy, in highly selected patients.

T4: Surgery with or without postoperative radiotherapy or definitive radiation therapy with surgery for salvage of radiation failures. Concomitant chemotherapy and radiation therapy with laryngectomy in patients who show a poor response to chemotherapy. This option has been used in highly selected patients.

In all patients with supraglottic tumors the neck should be electively treated even if it is clinically N0. Occult metastases are found in neck dissection specimens more commonly in patients with supraglottic carcinoma than in the other laryngeal subsites. This has been linked to T stage, in T1/T2 tumors; occult metastases are present in approximately 16% of the specimens. In T3/T4 tumors they are found in as many as 50% of the cases. Several institutions are now recommending bilateral neck dissections in patients with clinically N0 supraglottic cancer.

The 5-year survival of supraglottic tumors varies from 70% to 90% for stage I and stage II disease, falling to 40–60% for stage III disease and is as low as 10–45% for stage IV disease.

2.5.2　Glottic tumors
Mike Thomas and Tim Price

PRESENTATION

The cardinal symptom of glottic cancer is hoarseness and all patients with hoarseness that persists for longer than four to six weeks should be referred for evaluation of the larynx. Shortness of breath and stridor occur with large lesions and ulceration, and bleeding from an exophytic lesion can lead to hemoptysis. Sore throat and otalgia (ear ache) are ominous signs and usually only occur in advanced disease with supraglottic and tongue base involvement. Nodal metastases are uncommon especially in early stage disease due to the paucity of lymphatics in the glottis.

EPIDEMIOLOGY

The age group most commonly affected is 50–70 years with the male to female ratio of 5:1. The vast majority of glottis cancers are squamous cell carcinomas (SCC) and are as a result of the chronic consumption of tobacco and/or alcohol. However, glottic SCCs can occur in certain genetically predisposed individuals in the absence of tobacco smoke. Verrucous carcinomas are a highly differentiated variant of SCC and account for approximately 1–2% of vocal fold tumors.

CLINICAL APPEARANCE

The appearance of vocal cord tumors ranges from a nodule or thickening of a cord to areas of leukoplakia or laryngeal hyperkeratosis (Figs. 2.5.2.1 & 2.5.2.2) to raised, warty lesions or frank ulceration on one vocal cord. More advanced tumors will spread across the anterior commissure to involve the contralateral vocal cord or down into the subglottis or upward to involve the false cords and the supraglottis (Fig. 2.5.2.3). It is important to ascertain whether there is normal movement of the cord as fixation of the cord implies advanced disease (T3–4). The whole of the larynx including the subglottis as well as the postcricoid and upper esophagus should be evaluated (Video 5). The findings will allow accurate staging of the lesion and exclude a synchronous second primary tumor (1–5%). Adequate biopsies should be taken once the lesion has been fully assessed so as not to obscure further visualization with blood (Video 7) Fig. 2.5.2.4 & 2.5.2.5.

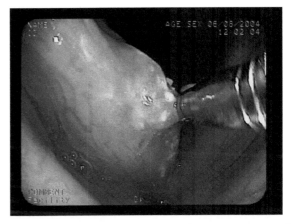

Figure 2.5.2.2 Biopsy being taken from the lesion. T1 squamous cell carcinoma.

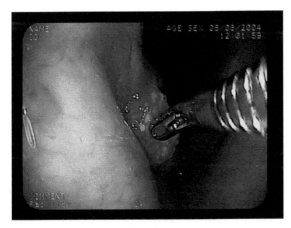

Figure 2.5.2.1 Leukoplakia of middle and anterior third of right vocal cord.

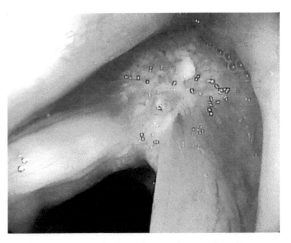

Figure 2.5.2.3 Anterior commissure squamous cell carcinoma.

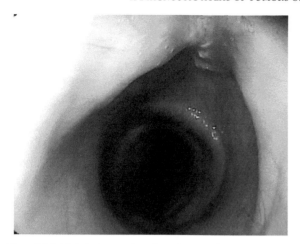

Figure 2.5.2.4 Subglottic extension of anterior commissure squamous cell carcinoma.

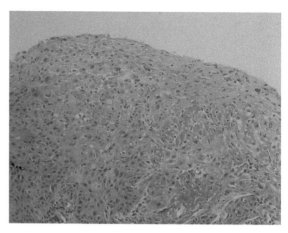

Figure 2.5.2.5 Laryngeal squamous mucosa with severe dysplasia and transition into moderately well differentiated squamous cell carcinoma (H&E, x200).

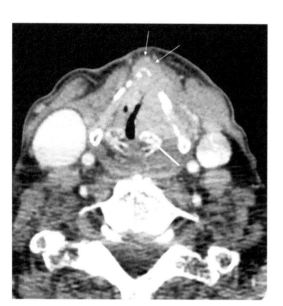

Figure 2.5.2.6 Postcontrast axial CT scan at level of true cord. Bulky soft tissue mass centered on left vocal cord crossing the midline anteriorly. Extralaryngeal spread through thyroid cartilage. Sclerotic left arytenoid. Arrows = extralaryngeal spread through thyroid cartilage. Thick arrow = sclerotic arytenoid.

IMAGING

Radiological investigations include a chest radiograph to check for lung metastases or a lung primary. A chest CT scan may be indicated if suspected lung metastases need further evaluation. A CT or MRI scan of the neck and larynx will help identify any impalpable lymph nodes and assess the extent of any laryngeal cartilage involvement (Figs 2.5.2.6 & 2.5.2.7).

The clinical and radiological findings allow the surgeon to stage the lesion using the TNM staging system, and the treatment offered depends on the stage (Video 8).

STAGING

TX: Primary tumor cannot be assessed.

T0: No evidence of primary tumor.

Tis: Carcinoma *in situ.*

T1: Tumor limited to the vocal cord(s) (may involve anterior or posterior commissure) with normal mobility.

T1a: Tumor limited to one vocal cord.

T1b: Tumor involves both vocal cords.

T2: Tumor extends to supraglottis and/or subglottis, or with impaired vocal cord mobility.

T3: Tumor limited to larynx with vocal cord fixation.

T4a: Tumor invades cricoid or thyroid cartilage and/or invades beyond the larynx (e.g., trachea, soft tissues of the neck including deep extrinsic muscles of the tongue, strap muscles, thyroid, or esophagus).

T4b: Tumor invades the prevertebral space, encases the carotid artery, or invades mediastinal structures.

MANAGEMENT

Treatment is either palliative or curative in intent depending on the stage of the disease and the patient's overall level of fitness.

Tis: There is evidence that this condition is reversible on smoking cessation. The entire mucosal abnormality will need to be excised to diagnose and differentiate it from invasive carcinoma. Excision biopsy is therefore a treatment of choice with a cure rate of around 90%. There are equal efficacy rates between surgical stripping and radiotherapy; there is however a 10% failure rate with primary radiotherapy. For recurrent disease endoscopic and conservative surgical removal are options as is radiotherapy.

T1: Single-modality treatment is recommended in the United Kingdom. Lesions are usually treated with radiotherapy with cure rates in excess of 90%. Small tumors confined to one vocal cord can be treated with endoscopic laser resection, giving

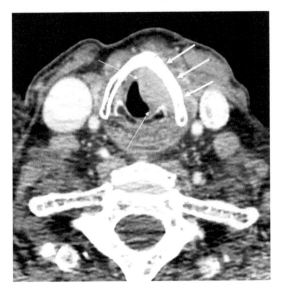

Figure 2.5.2.7 Postcontrast axial CT scan just below level of true cords. Subglottic extension of tumour (*thin arrows*). Note sclerotic left thyroid lamina (*thick arrows*). Arrows = subglottic extension.

similar results and allowing the surgeon to keep radiotherapy in reserve for possible recurrences. Open resection with a partial laryngectomy is also an option.

T2: Tumors are usually managed by radiotherapy or partial endoscopic laryngectomy with the laser in selected patients. Open organ preservation surgery is also an option; in unfavorable cases concurrent chemoradiation therapy has been used.

T3: Tumors are usually treated with radiotherapy but the results of salvage surgery for recurrences after radiotherapy are poor. High-volume tumors should be treated with primary surgery (laryngectomy and bilateral neck dissection) and postoperative radiotherapy.

T4: These tumors are treated via total laryngectomy and a bilateral neck dissection with postoperative radiotherapy. In selected patients concurrent chemoradiation therapy has been used to preserve laryngeal function.

Early glottic lesions rarely metastasize to cervical nodes and should raise the possibility of understaging. In treating the neck, levels II, III, IV, and V should be considered.

The overall 5-year survival for early glottic tumors is between 85% and 90%. Early T1 tumors, with no nodal involvement, do extremely well. Survival figures drop to 65–70% for stage III disease and are as low as 20% for stage IV disease.

2.5.3 Subglottic tumors
Mike Thomas

PRESENTATION

The difficulty in presentation is distinguishing between a true subglottic tumor and a spread into the subglottis from a glottic tumor. Dyspnea, with stridor is the main presenting symptom but hoarseness is present in approximately 30% of cases due to vocal fold fixation. Hemoptysis and cough are uncommon symptoms. Early tracheal obstruction can occur, necessitating either a tracheostomy or endoscopic debulking. Up to 20% of true subglottic tumors have evidence of cervical lymph-node metastases. Subglottic tumors spread to level VI (the pretracheal, Delphian node, in the central neck compartment) or to the paratracheal nodes in level VII (superior mediastinal and tracheoesphageal groove). In advanced disease the incidence of nodes can be as high as 50%. Mediastinal nodes can be involved in up to 46% of cases.

EPIDEMIOLOGY

Subglottic tumors are exceedingly rare accounting for less than 5% of all laryngeal cancers (Video 9). These are more common in men, presenting usually in the 6th or 7th decades. Most of them are squamous cell in origin; nonsquamous tumors arise from salivary gland tissue and neuroendocrine cells. Among salivary gland tumors adenocarcinoma is the commonest, but two-thirds of laryngeal adenoid cystic carcinomas occur in the subglottis with an equal male-to-female distribution. The most common sarcomas are the chondrosarcoma that usually arises from the posterior lamina of the cricoid cartilage. Tumors arising from neural crest cells include paragangliomas and carcinoid tumors; lymphomas and metastases have also been described.

CLINICAL APPEARANCE

The appearance is usually that of a smooth submucosal mass visible when the growth reaches the edge of the vocal fold or as a swelling below the anterior commissure (Fig. 2.5.3.1). Lesions can be bilateral and circumferential. The cricoid cartilage is involved early, as there is no intervening muscular layer to protect the cricoid. Partial or complete fixation of one or both vocal folds is common due to submucosal spread, superiorly, through the conus elasticus and can make differentiation between a true subglottic tumor and spread from a glottic tumor difficult. The hypopharynx and esophagus may be involved by posterior spread beneath the cricoid cartilage. Early stage T1 and T2 tumors are not common, around 20% of cases, but if found, usually do not have nodal disease. 80% of cases are stage T3–T4 at presentation. It is important to assess the entire larynx including the hypopharynx and upper esophagus together with the trachea.

IMAGING

Radiological investigations include a chest radiograph for lung metastases and to exclude a lung primary; if metastases are shown or if suspicion is high, a CT scan of the chest is warranted.

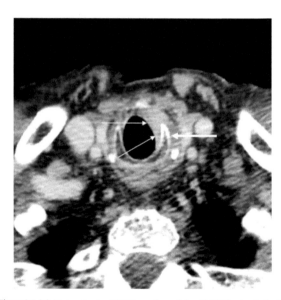

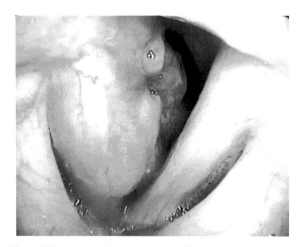

Figure 2.5.3.1 A large subglottic squamous cell carcinoma invading upward into the right vocal cord. Superior surface of the cord largely unaffected by tumor.

Figure 2.5.3.2 Postcontrast axial CT scan through hyoid. Thickening in the left subglottic region. Subtle sclerosis of the adjacent cricoid. Arrows = subglottic tumor. Thick arrow = sclerotic cricoid cartilage.

An accurate assessment of the anatomical extent of the tumor is needed. A CT scan will include the larynx to assess invasion of cricoid and thyroid cartilages and extension through cricothyroid membrane into anterior soft tissues of the neck and thyroid gland. An MRI scan may be needed if there is any doubt about soft-tissue resolution and may help with cartilage invasion. Both are excellent at assessing subglottic extension but MRI will provide sagittal images. An accurate radiological assessment of cervical node involvement including levels VI and VII is essential. The clinical and radiological findings allow accurate staging of the lesion with the help of the TNM staging system and allow planning for treatment (Fig. 2.5.3.2).

STAGING

TX: Primary tumor cannot be assessed.

T0: No evidence of primary tumor.

Tis: Carcinoma *in situ*.

T1: Tumor limited to subglottis.

T2: Tumor extends to vocal cord(s) with normal or impaired mobility.

T3: Tumor limited to larynx with vocal cord fixation.

T4a: Tumor invades through cricoid or thyroid cartilage and/or invades tissues beyond the larynx, e.g., trachea, soft tissues of neck, thyroid and/or esophagus.

T4b: Tumor invades prevertebral space or mediastinal structures, or encases the carotid artery.

MANAGEMENT

It is difficult to give an accurate review of the treatment options as these are rare tumors and there are no large series available to give meaningful comparisons. Due to late presentation the overall survival is low, 25% at three years.

T1 and T2 lesions: Although rare, are usually treated with radical radiotherapy to the larynx, upper trachea, paratracheal, and superior mediastinal nodes. Due to the change in contour from the neck to the thorax, this is a relatively difficult area to irradiate. Some centers have used partial laryngectomy for early stage disease (stage I–II).

T3: Total laryngectomy and neck dissection, usually bilateral to include levels VI and VII and ipsilateral or a total thyroidectomy followed up by postoperative radiotherapy.

T4: Total laryngectomy and neck dissection, usually bilateral to include levels VI and VII and ipsilateral or a total thyroidectomy followed up by postoperative radiotherapy.

Some centers are using simultaneous chemotherapy and hyperfractionated radiation therapy for advanced stage disease.

2.6.1 Hypopharynx tumors
Tom Wilson

The hypopharynx is the lowest region of the pharynx situated between the oropharynx and the esophagus. Its upper limit is the hyoid and the lower limit is the lower margin of the cricoid cartilage. It is conventionally subdivided into three anatomical areas: posterior pharyngeal wall, pyriform fossa, and postcricoid region. The hypopharynx lies behind and lateral to the larynx but does not include it.

PRESENTATION

Most of the tumors occurring in the hypopharynx are squamous cell carcinomas, followed by minor salivary gland carcinomas or other soft tissue sarcomas. Tumors are most commonly found in the pyriform fossa (70%). They tend to present late and have a tendency to spread within the mucosa beneath an intact epidermis by invasion of the lymphatic tissues giving rise to "skip" lesions. Hypopharyngeal carcinoma is thus associated with a particularly high rate of nodal metastases and second primary (synchronous) tumors at presentation. The tumor can also spread to other head and neck subsites via the paralaryngeal spaces. Symptoms include a vague sensation of a lump in the throat, food sticking, constitutional upset, and classically an unrelenting otalgia if the glossopharyngeal nerve is involved by a tumor in the pyriform fossa. Signs include pooling of saliva in the hypopharynx (Chevalier Jackson's sign Fig. 2.6.1.1) and a directly palpable neck mass.

EPIDEMIOLOGY

More than 95% of tumors of the hypopharynx are SCC; yet it is rarer than other head and neck SCCs with incidence in the United States of 0.7/100,000 per year and a mortality rate of 0.1/100,000. It tends to be a disease of the elderly and affects men more than women (2:1) with the commonest presentation being a male in his 70s. The associated risk factors depend upon the subsite of the hypopharynx involved. Most hypopharyngeal tumors are associated with chronic tobacco use, betel nut chewing, and excessive alcohol consumption. Tumors of the postcricoid appear to be associated with gross nutritional deficiencies and in particular with Plummer–Vinson syndrome.

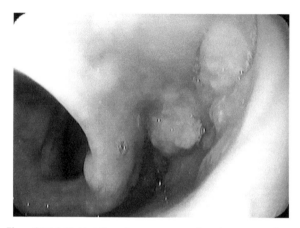

Figure 2.6.1.2 Right piriform fossa squamous cell carcinoma presenting as multiple submucosal lesions.

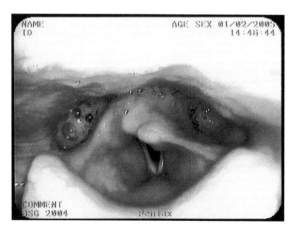

Figure 2.6.1.1 Pooling of saliva in left and right pyriform fossa after swallowing (Chevalier Jackson's sign).

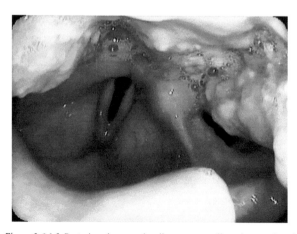

Figure 2.6.1.3 Posterior pharyngeal wall squamous cell carcinoma viewed from the level of epiglottis. Lesion spreads inferiorly to the level of the arytenoids but not involving piriform fossa or postcricoid area.

CLINICAL APPEARANCE

Hypopharyngeal tumors tend to present late and are in an area of the upper aero-digestive tract that is difficult to visualize in the clinic. They are usually seen when performing a pharyngoscopy under general anesthetic for investigation of suspicious symptoms or following a suspicious appearance on flexible laryngoscopy. Pyriform fossa tumors usually appear as plaque-like lesions with raised edges and superficial ulceration (Fig. 2.6.1.2). Posterior pharyngeal wall carcinomas tend to be larger and exophytic (Fig. 2.6.1.3). Care must be taken to assess the rest of the larynx and proximal esophagus to rule out invasion of the larynx and synchronous second primaries or skip lesions. The neck must be thoroughly examined as most patients will have either the primary tumor palpable as a neck mass or will have palpable nodal disease.

IMAGING

SCC of the hypopharynx has a particular tendency for late presentation along with nodal metastases and synchronous aero-digestive tract malignancy. It is important to image patients with this in mind so imaging of the neck and chest, with MRI and/or CT, allowing the staging of the disease prior to treatment planning is mandatory. Patients are at risk of aspiration so a chest x-ray is indicated for that reason alone. If the esophagus has not been assessed by endoscopy it should be imaged by a barium swallow.

STAGING

T1: Tumor limited to 1 subsite of the hypopharynx and ≤2 cm in greatest dimension

T2: Tumor invades more than 1 subsite of the hypopharynx or an adjacent site, or measures >2 cm but ≤4 cm in greatest diameter without fixation of hemilarynx

T3: Tumor measures >4 cm in greatest dimension or with fixation of hemilarynx

T4a: Tumor invades thyroid/cricoid cartilage, hyoid bone, thyroid gland, esophagus, or central compartment soft tissue, which includes prelaryngeal strap muscles and subcutaneous fat

T4b: Tumor invades prevertebral fascia, encases the carotid artery, or involves mediastinal structures

MANAGEMENT

Management of SCC of the hypopharynx will depend upon the disease stage and the exact site of the primary tumor. Early-stage disease (T1 or T2 with no clinical evidence of neck metastases) is very rare and, unfortunately, most patients present with advanced-stage disease (III or IV). Advanced-stage disease is associated with delayed presentation, regional metastases, and significant patient comorbidity, ultimately leading to a poor prognosis. These all factor in the treatment planning but often dictate that treatment is with a palliative intent. In a suitable case, the primary site can be treated with curative intent by either surgery (usually a laryngopharyngectomy) or radiotherapy. But surgical resection of the disease may be compromised by the need to obtain clear surgical margins and resulting functional compromise. Surgical resection may be supplemented by reconstruction as necessary, with an esophageal reconstruction or a gastric pull-up needed if a significant resection of pharyngeal mucosa or esophagus has taken place. As a general rule all patients need regional neck nodes treated by either surgery or radiotherapy bilaterally. If the neck and primary site are treated by primary surgery then the patient will be recommended for postoperative radiotherapy with concomitant chemotherapy (cisplatin).

2.6.2 Pyriform fossa tumors
Hemi Patel

PRESENTATION

Pyriform fossa tumors present late, in fact T1 N0 cases (see staging) represent only 2% of the cases seen and stage III, 70%. Neck node involvement is high, occurring in up to 75% of cases with 10% being bilateral at presentation and distant metastasis rates are the highest of any cancers in this region. Patients may present with chronic sore throat, dysphagia, foreign body or globus sensation, and referred otalgia. A painless lump in the neck is the only symptom in up to 20% of patients. Late symptoms include hemoptysis, hoarseness of voice, halitosis, and weight loss.

EPIDEMIOLOGY

Pyriform fossa cancers represent approximately 7% of all cancers of the upper aero-digestive tract and 70% of all hypopharyngeal cancers.

Men are much more commonly affected than women and are typically 55–70 years of age at presentation.

Risk factors for the development of pyriform fossa squamous cell carcinoma (SCC) as with larynx and other sites in the pharynx include tobacco smoking, alcohol ingestion, diet lacking in fresh fruit and vegetables, gastroesophageal reflux disease, and HPV 16 seropositivity.

It is interesting to note that people on a good Mediterranean diet have less than half the risk of developing pharyngeal cancers and that a high intake of red meat, processed meat, and fried foods increases the risk of pharyngeal cancer.

HISTOPATHOLOGY AND CLINICAL APPEARANCE

Ninety percent of the cancers in this area are SCCs. The vast majority are poorly differentiated. Tumors are mostly advanced at presentation and an obvious lesion is apparent. This can vary macroscopically from a mucosal ulcer to a large exophytic mass. On occasion only subtle signs are present, such as submucosal fullness (skip lesions) or pooling of saliva (Jackson's sign) (Figs. 2.6.2.1–2.6.2.3).

IMAGING AND WORKUP

All patients should undergo a thorough endoscopic evaluation of the larynx, pharynx, and esophagus in order to obtain tissue specimens for histology and for clinical staging. Ten percent of patients will have a second primary tumor at presentation and have a lifetime risk of developing a second primary of 20%. They therefore need a careful long-term follow-up.

CT scan and MRI are used to evaluate the primary tumor and regional lymph nodes. They are complementary and demonstrate accurately the tumor size, site, and its involvement with the surrounding tissue (Figs. 2.6.2.4 & 2.6.2.5).

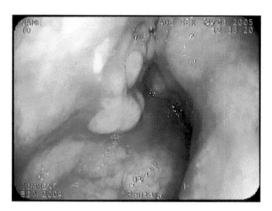

Figure 2.6.2.1 Right pyriform fossa submucosal squamous cell carcinoma (skip lesions).

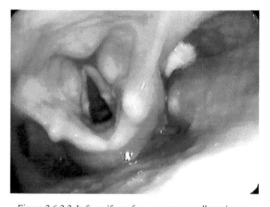

Figure 2.6.2.2 Left pyriform fossa squamous cell carcinoma.

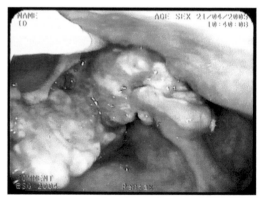

Figure 2.6.2.3 Stage 4 disease with spread to the arytenoids bilaterally and right aryepiglottic fold. Feeding tube *in situ.*

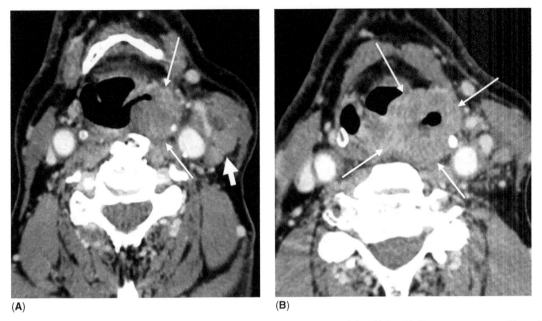

(A)   **(B)**

Figure 2.6.2.4 A 83-year-old male with dysphagia. Left pyriform fossa squamous cell carcinoma. (A) and (B) Axial CT scans post contrast of hypopharynx. Circumferential thickening of the left pyriform fossa extending into the posterior pharyngeal wall (*arrows*). Enlarged left level 2/3 lymph node (*thick arrow*).

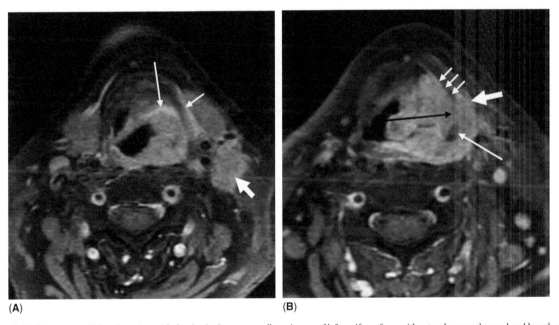

(A)   **(B)**

Figure 2.6.2.5 A 61-year-old female patient with dysphagia. Squamous cell carcinoma of left pyriform fossa with extrapharyngeal spread and lymph node metastasis. Axial fatsat T1 post-contrast images. (A) At the level of hyoid. Enhancing mass in the left pyriform fossa extending into the left vallecula (*arrow*) and infiltrating the left hyoid (*short arrow*). Level 2/3 lymph node (*thick arrow*). (B) At the level of thyroid cartilage. Infiltration of the left paraglottic fat (*short arrows*) with extension posterior to the left thyroid ala (*arrow*) and infiltration of the strap muscles (*thick arrow*). Note also infiltration of the left thyroid cartilage (*black arrow*).

Chest radiograph and chest CT will identify pulmonary metastasis or a second primary in the lungs.

STAGING

T Staging (Specific for Hypopharynx)

T1: Tumor ≤2 cm and limited to one subsite of hypopharynx

T2: Tumor >2 cm –4 cm or more than one subsite of hypopharynx

T3: Tumor >4 cm or with hemilarynx fixation

T4a: Involvement of thyroid or cricoid cartilage, hyoid bone, thyroid gland, esophagus, and central compartment soft tissue

T4b: Involvement of prevertebral fascia, carotid artery, and mediastinal structures

Stage groupings for oral cavity, oropharynx, hypopharynx, and laryngeal cancers are displayed in a table.

Stage I	T1	
Stage II	T2	
Stage III	T1,T2	N1
	T3	N0, N1
Stage IVA	T1, T2, T3	N2
	T4a	N0, N1, N2
Stage IVB	T4b	Any N
Stage IVC	Any T	Any N
	M1	

MANAGEMENT

Like other head and neck malignancies the treatment of pyriform fossa SCC is complex and must be individualized to the patient. The treatment varies from patient to patient depending on the stage of the disease, local expertise, the fitness of the patients and their wishes.

Early Cancer (Stage I and II)

Treatment option can be either radical external beam radiotherapy (EBR) with concomitant chemotherapy or conservative surgery with bilateral selective neck dissection.

Locally Advanced Cancer (Stage III and IV)

These patients may be treated with laryngopharyngectomy and reconstruction in suitably resectable cases; if this fails, an organ preservation approach using chemoradiotherapy with the option of salvage surgery is the next line of treatment.

In small tumors where there is sufficient residual pharyngeal mucosa primary closure is sometimes possible. In the rest, reconstruction of the defect with a myocutaneous flap is usually necessary. Commonly used approaches are the traditional pectoralis major pedicle flap or microvascular free flaps, such as the radial forearm or anterolateral thigh myocutaneous flaps. Choice of treatment depends on local expertise and the defect to be reconstructed. Some centers now advocate the routine use of flap reconstruction in postradiotherapy patients, citing lower rates of wound complications such as pharyngocutaneous fistula. Where there is involvement of the cervical esophagus then an esophagectomy is also performed with gastric interposition or a tubed jejunal free flap.

Regardless of the stage all patients should have some form of treatment to the neck due to the high incidence of occult metastasis. This may be by neck dissection or EBR.

Postoperative radiotherapy has been shown to improve locoregional control and survival where there is extracapsular spread or positive surgical margins.

OUTCOME AND PROGNOSIS

Stage I and II cancers have five-year survival rates approaching 70% and 30% in stage III and IV cancers.

2.6.3 Post cricoid tumors
Wyn Parry

PRESENTATION

Long duration (frequently 6 months plus) of often vague symptoms with insidious onset before a diagnosis is made is not uncommon. Presenting symptoms include a sensation of a foreign body in the throat or globus-type features. Dysphagia occurs later and is particularly ominous if accompanied by referred otalgia. Palpable neck masses due to lymph node metastases may be the presenting feature in 20% of patients, as may a hoarse voice either due to invasion of the posterior crico-arytenoids or a recurrent laryngeal nerve involvement.

EPIDEMIOLOGY

Tobacco use, often associated with excess alcohol consumption, is a common etiological factor. Previous radiotherapy may be relevant in a small number of patients. Plummer–Vinson syndrome is a classical association with postcricoid web formation.

Worldwide, there is a slight male preponderance in incidence, though in areas with higher incidences overall (United Kingdom, India), there is a more striking female:male ratio of 3:1, possibly reflecting differing frequencies of Plummer–Vinson syndrome.

HISTOLOGY AND CLINICAL APPEARANCE

Squamous cell carcinomas are overwhelmingly the most common histological group. Adenocarcinoma, sarcoma, and melanoma, though reported, are all very unusual. Submucosal spread, along with skip lesions are common.

Lymphatic spread is common; 75% of patients will have microscopic cervical nodal disease at presentation and 10% will have bilateral disease.

Postcricoid carcinomas are usually detected on transnasal laryngoesophagoscopy (TNLE) as irregular mucosal tumors often with an inflamed, haemorrhagic surface. A careful survey of the mucosa is necessary to assess for possible skip lesions (Figs. 2.6.3.1 & 2.6.3.2).

IMAGING

Contrast swallow may be helpful if carefully performed since small mucosal irregularities may be demonstrated. Interpretation is however difficult (Fig. 2.6.3.3).

CT scanning is particularly useful, both in terms of assessing local disease and also lymphatic and more distant spread. CT is usually able to allow assessment of, for example, cricoid invasion, extension into the cervical oesophagus, and tongue base involvement. CT is more limited in assessing tissue planes and particular muscle layer involvement, and MRI is more useful here (Figs. 2.6.3.4–2.6.3.6).

Endoscopy, including panendoscopy, is vital for tissue confirmation and assessment of resectability. A rigid bronchoscopy may be necessary to assess tracheal involvement.

STAGING
T Staging

TX: primary tumor cannot be assessed

T0: no evidence of primary tumor

Tis: Carcinoma *in situ*

T1: Tumor <2 cm

T2: Tumor >2 cm but <4 cm

T3: Tumor >4 cm but no fixation of hemilarynx

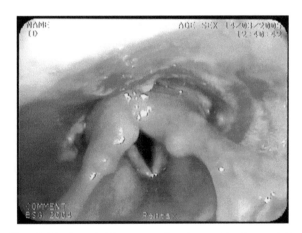

Figure 2.6.3.1 Post-cricoid squamous cell carcinoma with submucosal skip lesions in the right piriform fossa.

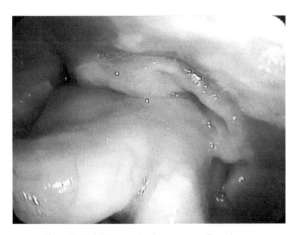

Figure 2.6.3.2 T4 postcricoid squamous cell carcinoma.

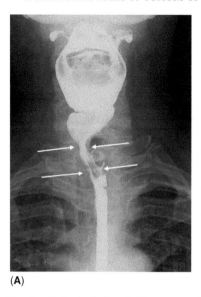
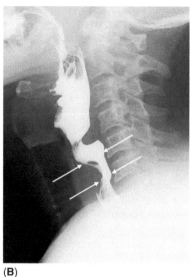

(A) **(B)**

Figure 2.6.3.3 A 66-year-old male with dysphagia. Postcricoid squamous cell carcinoma. (A) AP and (B) lateral barium swallow examination. Irregular stricture in the postcricoid esophagus (*arrows*).

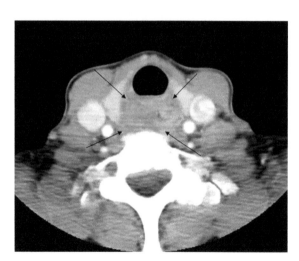

Figure 2.6.3.4 An axial post-intravenous contrast CT scan just below the level of cricoid cartilage. Eccentric thickening of postcricoid cervical esophagus (*arrows*).

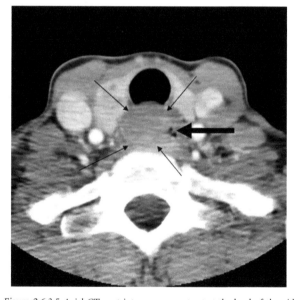

Figure 2.6.3.5 Axial CT post-intravenous contrast at the level of thyroid gland. Eccentric thickening of post-cricoid esophagus (*thin arrow*). Thick arrow = esophageal lumen.

T4a: Invasion of thyroid/cricoid cartilage, thyroid gland, strap muscles, or esophagus

T4b: Invasion of prevertebral fascia, carotid encasement

N Staging

NX: Regional nodes cannot be assessed

N0: No cervical nodes

N1: Single ipsilateral node <3 cm

N2: Single ipsilateral node >3 cm but <6 cm, or multiple ipsilateral nodes <6 cm, or bilateral nodes <6 cm

N3: Any node >6 cm

M Staging

MX: Distant metastases cannot be assessed

M0: No distant metastases

M1: Distant metastases present

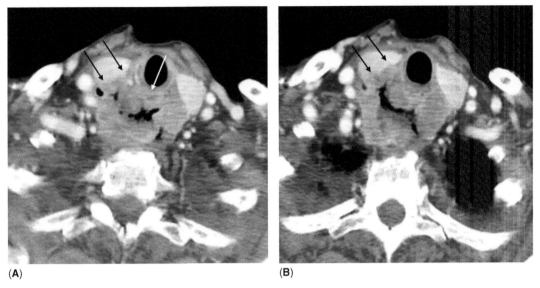

(A)   (B)

Figure 2.6.3.6 A 90-year-old female with 8 months' history of dysphagia. Large post-cricoid squamous cell carcinoma. Axial CT scans post contrast just above suprasternal notch. (A) and (B) Circumferential thickening of the post cricoid esophagus invading the right lobe of the thyroid (*black arrows*). Note also erosion of the posterior cricoid (*white arrow*).

MANAGEMENT

Optimal management involves surgical resection and adjuvant radiotherapy. The extent of any surgical resection is substantial in view of laryngeal involvement, the possibility of skip lesions and the requirement for clear resection margins. Unilateral or, usually bilateral neck dissections are likely to be indicated. Certainly for all cases with T2 or greater primary lesions, resection of the primary tumor will require a pharyngo-laryngo-esophagectomy with gastric mobilization and tube formation to allow the construction of a neo-esophagus which is anastomosed to the tongue base to restore continuity. Esophagectomy and gastric tube formation can be carried out transhiatally or via thoracotomy.

Alternative strategies include more localized tumor resection and interposition of a vascularized jejunal graft, or otherwise myocutaneous flap (deltopectoral or pectoralis major) reconstruction of the pharynx.

Apart from absolute contraindications to resection (carotid encasement, involvement of the prevertebral fascia/muscles, metastatic disease) surgery should be considered in all other suitable patients. Results with pharyngolaryngectomy and associated esophagectomy via left thoracotomy have been associated with 0% mortality, and certainly perioperative mortalities of <5–10% should be attainable in centers used to procedures of this complexity.

Five-year survival figures overall are 25–40%, with 48% for T1, 23% T2, 5% T3, and <2% T4. With added N1 disease in the T1/T2 group, the five-year survival is halved.

Small (T1/2) primary tumors may be treated with radiotherapy alone especially if, due to related comorbidities (which can be considerable in this group) radical surgery represents an unacceptable risk to the individual patient.

2.7 Esophageal tumors
Wyn Parry and Tim Price

PRESENTATION
Esophageal carcinoma may present to the ENT surgeon in several ways, including dysphagia (usually progressive for solids, then liquids), odynophagia, globus symptoms in the neck or upper chest, or even acutely with a food bolus obstruction. The level at which symptoms occur, particularly dysphagia, rarely correlates with the level of any pathology except perhaps in high cervical tumors. Recurrent laryngeal nerve involvement as an isolated entity and its presentation are uncommon except in advanced stages of the disease.

EPIDEMIOLOGY
Most commonly encountered in male patients with a peak incidence at age 50–70, although the mean age is declining as the incidence slowly rises. Risk factors include smoking, obesity, and excess alcohol consumption. Prolonged reflux of acid, bile, and gastric content may lead to progressive metaplasia of the esophageal mucosa (Barrett's esophagus) with an eventual dysplastic change (Fig. 2.7.1). Progressive dysplasia, especially when severe on histological grounds (cellular atypia, nuclear changes) may be the precursor of adenocarcinoma in many, perhaps the majority, of the patients. Other etiologies are much less common, including achalasia and Plummer–Vinson syndrome. There is an increase of esophageal cancers in patients who have a history of previous upper aero-digestive malignancies.

HISTOLOGY AND CLINICAL APPEARANCE
Most carcinomas will occur at or around the gastroesophageal junction or distal esophagus, and adenocarcinoma is the most common type both here and overall (Fig. 2.7.2). Squamous carcinomas tend to occur in the upper esophagus (Fig. 2.7.3), this group including the postcricoid carcinomas.

The pooling of saliva in both pyriform fossae (Jackson's sign) is a good indication of a lesion in the proximal esophagus or postcricoid area (Fig. 2.6.1.1 in chap. 2.6.1). Many lesions will be ulcerative or polypoid in appearance on gross inspection, but submucosal infiltration is well recognized and can be difficult to assess on endoscopy. Large lesions may narrow the lumen of the esophagus with a complete loss of the normal folds in the mucosa (Figs. 2.7.4–2.7.6).

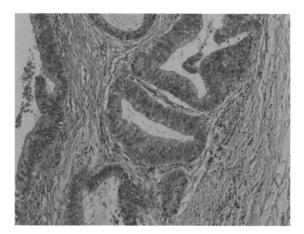

Figure 2.7.2 Mucosa containing malignant glands, characterized by hyperchromasia, loss of nuclear polarity, and desmoplastic stromal reaction, all diagnostic of an esophageal adenocarcinoma.

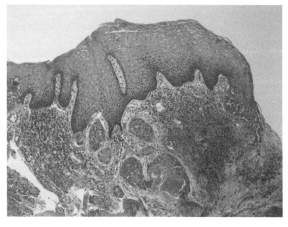

Figure 2.7.3 Esophageal mucosa lined with hyperplastic squamous epithelium and underneath, a growth of a moderately to well-differentiated, partly keratinizing invasive squamous cell carcinoma (H&E, x200).

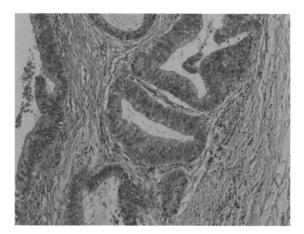

Figure 2.7.1 Barrett's esophagus- confluent metaplastic changes secondary to acid reflux.

Tumors in the upper third and particularly those in relation to the carina may impinge on or invade the airway, sometimes resulting in fistula formation. A rigid bronchoscopy is mandatory in assessing such proximal tumors to exclude airway involvement.

IMAGING

Contrast swallow may show an irregular mucosal pattern with narrowing of the lumen (the so-called "apple core lesion" (Fig. 2.7.7A & B) and proximal dilatation, but endoscopy is mandatory for a detailed assessment of tumor location and length as well as obtaining biopsies for tissue diagnosis.

Endoscopic ultrasound (EUS) may be useful in assessing tumor depth, including involvement of extraesophageal tissues including the aorta and pericardium on occasions, as well as possibly assessing local nodal disease.

A CT scan is required to assess likely sites of nodal (local, regional and distant) spread as well as more distant metastatic disease to extraesophageal sites (liver, lungs, bone). PET scanning may also be helpful in this assessment.

STAGING

T-Staging

X: Tumor cannot be assessed

0: No tumor is evident

Is: *In-situ* carcinoma

Does not breach submucosa

Spreads not beyond lamina propria

Invades paraesophageal tissues but not adjacent structures

Adjacent structures invaded

N-Staging

X: Nodes cannot be assessed

0: No regional node metastases

1: Regional node metastases

M-Staging

X: Metastases cannot be assessed

0: No metastatic disease present

1: Metastatic disease present, including distal nodal groups

Stage	TNM	5-year survival (%)
I	T1, N0, M0	60
II	T2/T3, N0	20
	T1/T2, N1	
III	T3, N1	<10
	T4, any N, M0	
IV	Any T, any N, M1	<1

MANAGEMENT

Very early tumors may be suitable for laser resection, photodynamic therapy (PDT), or endoscopic mucosal resection, though the numbers of patients seen with this type of disease are very small.

In practice, most patients will present with more advanced disease and, while resection offers the best prognosis, the majority of patients will have inoperable disease due to either a local extension or a distant metastatic spread. Stage of disease and fitness of the patient are thus the principal considerations in selecting appropriate treatment options. Current evidence indicates an improved prognosis with neoadjuvant chemotherapy prior to surgery, at least for the majority of mid/distal third tumors. Radical radiotherapy may occasionally be curative especially in small, localized tumors in patients too unfit for resection.

A resection with an immediate reconstruction of the upper GI tract using stomach, colon, or small bowel (in that order of preference) is the surgical aim.

Palliative interventions are frequently necessary, either at presentation or during/after treatment. These include laser ablation, external beam radiotherapy, brachytherapy, tumor dilation, and stent insertion. Palliative resection should not be offered to patients with advanced disease, and tumor bypass procedures such as cervical esophagostomy and feeding gastrostomy/jejunostomy though theoretical options require careful judgment in their use.

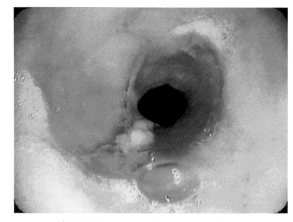

Figure 2.7.4 An early mid-esophageal carcinoma.

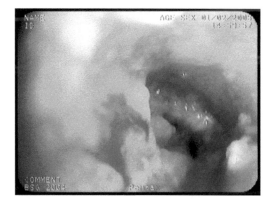

Figure 2.7.5 An advanced circumferential esophageal tumor. Almost complete obstruction with a very small lumen present. Area of bleeding from which biopsy was taken in the clinic.

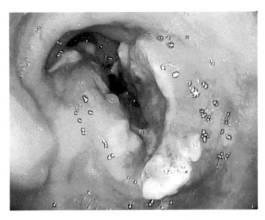

Figure 2.7.6 An advanced obstructing squamous cell carcinoma at 27 cm.

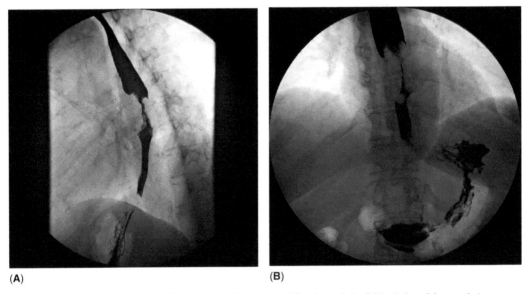

(A)   **(B)**

Figure 2.7.7 (A) A lateral view of barium swallow showing typical "apple core lesion." (B) AP view of the same lesion.

2.9 Tumors of the thyroid
Don J. Premachandra

INTRODUCTION
Thyroid tumors present as midline swellings in the neck. When the thyroid enlarges to double its normal size it is usually referred to as a goiter. The vast majority of thyroid swellings are benign. They usually present as nodular enlargement and can be detected by palpation. The incidence of thyroid nodules in the general adult population is around 10% in women and 2% in men. However, if examined by ultrasound, the incidence can go up to 50%.

PRESENTATION AND EPIDEMIOLOGY
Goiters are commonly found, but malignant tumors of the thyroid are uncommon. They have an incidence of 3.5 per 100,000 in women and 1.3 per 100,000 in men. Thyroid cancer is the commonest malignant endocrine tumor, but only represents 1% of all malignancies. Although the exact etiology of the thyroid cancer is not known, populations exposed to ionizing radiation, for example Hiroshima and Chernobyl, have a higher incidence of papillary carcinoma. Medullary carcinoma can present with multiple endocrine neoplasia [multiple endocrine neoplasia (MEN) syndromes].

MALIGNANT TUMORS OF THE THYROID
For clinical evaluation, treatment, and prognosis thyroid carcinoma is divided into two main histological types:

Well-differentiated thyroid carcinoma (good prognosis):

- Papillary carcinoma 80–85%
- Follicular carcinoma 10–15%

Poorly differentiated thyroid carcinoma (poor prognosis):

- Anaplastic carcinoma 1%
- Hurthle cell carcinoma

In addition to these two categories, medullary carcinoma constitutes 5–10% of thyroid cancer, which has a fair prognosis, especially when treated aggressively at an early stage.

CLINICAL PRESENTATION
Tumors usually present with a simple nodule in the thyroid gland. Large benign swellings of the thyroid gland can cause airway obstruction, especially when there is gross enlargement and a retrosternal extension (Fig. 2.9.1). Multinodular goiters are slow-growing and almost always benign. Swellings, which are hard and present with rapid growth, hoarseness of voice, dysphagia, and cervical lymphadenopathy, should arouse a strong suspicion of malignancy. Family history of thyroid malignancy and exposure to radiation should be elicited in the history.

EXAMINATION
The most important part of the clinical evaluation of thyroid lumps is to exclude malignancy. Benign goiters and those genuine retrosternal goiters that have the potential to cause airway obstruction may need elective surgical removal. If these patients present with acute airway obstruction, emergency endotracheal intubation as well as tracheostomy can be extremely difficult.

Single solitary solid nodules, which are usually follicular adenomas, have a 10% chance of being malignant. In addition to palpation of the thyroid, the rest of the neck should be examined for enlarged cervical lymph nodes. Those thyroid masses in which it is not possible to palpate the lower margin may have an extension into the chest to become retrosternal goiters. If the retrosternal component does not rise into the neck on swallowing and they develop hyperemia of skin with engorgement of neck veins on raising the arms above the head (Pemberton's sign), they may have a large retrosternal component. It is essential to record the function of the vocal cords, which in turn, gives the state of the recurrent laryngeal nerve (RLN).

INVESTIGATIONS
The assessment of thyroid hormone levels determines the biochemical state of the gland. Thyroid antibodies are raised in conditions like thyroiditis, which can mimic malignant tumors due to the hard nature of the gland as well as the presence of cervical lymph nodes.

The most important investigation is the fine needle aspiration for cytology (FNAC) of the thyroid mass. Those nodules, which are difficult to palpate, or have poor aspirates, which are

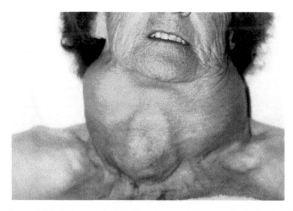

Figure 2.9.1 Patient with thyroid goiter for 30 years who had refused surgery. Presented with a sudden enlargement of thyroid and breathing difficulties. Histology subsequently revealed malignant transformation (follicular carcinoma).

insufficient for diagnosis, should be further investigated with ultra sound-guided FNAC.

Retrosternal goiters may need CT scans without intravenous contrast if malignancy is suspected. Giving radioactive iodine contrast can cause a delay in treatment with radioactive iodine if the tumor is found to be malignant.

If there is any suspicion of a lymphoma of the thyroid, a core biopsy is often sufficient to make a histological diagnosis. Failing this, a small incision biopsy is not contraindicated. A similar strategy can be employed to make a diagnosis of anaplastic carcinoma. All the patients diagnosed with medullary carcinoma should be further investigated to exclude multiple endocrine neoplasias.

TREATMENT

Treatment for a well-differentiated thyroid cancer is total thyroidectomy, followed by radio iodine treatment. Papillary carcinoma, which tends to produce lymph node metastases, needs a selective block dissection of the neck. Follicular carcinoma is unlikely to produce lymph node metastases.

Medullary carcinoma needs a more aggressive surgical treatment. In addition to a total thyroidectomy, it needs a prophylactic neck dissection, as the tumor is not radiosensitive.

Patients with MEN syndromes with positive RET gene need a prophylactic total thyroidectomy. Anaplastic thyroid cancers usually occur in the extreme old age and tend to present with wide local and systemic spread not amenable to any rational surgical treatment and tend to succumb within 2–6 months. If the tumor is confined to the gland without systemic spread, they can be treated with total thyroidectomy, which may prolong the survival period.

SURGICAL REMOVAL OF THE THYROID GLAND

When total thyroidectomy is carried out for malignant thyroid tumors it is most important to preserve RLNs as well as the parathyroid glands. Surgeons should be able to identify the RLNs as intracapsular resection may not be adequate to clear the margins. The old textbooks that advocate the ligation of the inferior thyroid arteries lateral to RLNs as one main branch should be ignored to preserve the blood supply to the parathyroid glands. Instead, branches of the inferior thyroid artery should be ligated individually so as to preserve the branches to the parathyroid glands. All efforts should be made to preserve the RLNs, especially when the preoperative function is normal. There is very little to gain by sacrificing the nerve in order to get clear margins, as the few remaining cancer cells can be mopped up by radio iodine therapy.

The use of intraoperative nerve monitoring should be encouraged and should be used by all. There is a misconception in some surgeons that the nerve monitor is used for identification of the nerve and therefore it is not necessary for experienced surgeons to use it. The real reason for its use is the confirmation of definitive identification and preservation of the nerve function at the end of the procedure. Modern nerve monitors can record the function of the nerve, which may be of use in medicolegal situations (Figs. 2.9.2–2.9.4).

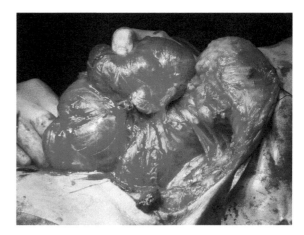

Figure 2.9.3 Left lobe of the thyroid dissected away from the recurrent laryngeal nerve seen crossing the trachea in the center of the picture.

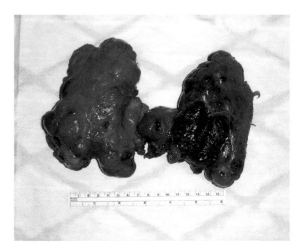

Figure 2.9.4 A surgical specimen.

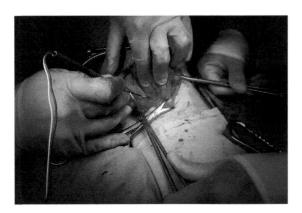

Figure 2.9.2 Identifying the recurrent laryngeal nerve during a surgery.

PROGNOSIS

Well-differentiated thyroid carcinoma has an excellent prognosis. There are large numbers of patients who survive with recurrences without succumbing to the disease. Female patients who are between 15 and 45 years have a good prognosis, especially when diagnosed at an early stage. Male patents and those who develop carcinoma in the extremes of life have a poor prognosis. Anaplastic carcinoma has an extremely poor prognosis.

TREATMENT OF RECURRENT DISEASE

Those patients with radio iodine sensitive recurrences are usually treated with radioactive iodine. External beam radiation, though used, has limited value. Surgical excision can be challenging as recurrences are usually close to the RLNs and any damage to them results in hoarseness of voice and if bilateral, a tracheostomy. If these complications occur, the treatment may seem to the patient, to be worse than living with a slow growing recurrence.

3.1 Benign nasopharyngeal tumors
Hemi Patel

PRESENTATION

Benign tumors of the nasopharynx are rare, they can arise from all constituent elements, and so various epithelial, mesenchymal, fibro-osseous, neurogenic, and vascular tumors have been described in the literature (Figs. 3.1.1 & 3.1.2). The most common acquired tumors amongst these are the simple squamous papilloma, juvenile angiofibroma, and benign salivary gland tumors. The most common developmental tumors are gliomas, cephaloceles, and a Rathke pouch cyst.

They present with nasal obstruction, epistaxis, nasal discharge, and hyposmia. Non-nasal symptoms include otalgia, hearing loss (glue ear), headache, facial swelling, and trismus.

IMAGING AND WORKUP

CT and MRI are complementary modalities in the diagnosis and evaluation of tumor extent.

CT details bone, foramina, and osteogenic lesions while MRI accurately delineates soft tissue structures and lesions.

Angiography is indicated in tumors suspected to be highly vascular, and can be combined with preoperative embolization when surgery is indicated in hypervascular tumors such as juvenile angiofibroma.

In many cases clinical presentation and imaging provide sufficient information for diagnosis and treatment planning. Where there is doubt, endoscopic biopsy is indicated.

TREATMENT

The treatment of choice for a vast majority of benign nasopharyngeal tumors is surgical excision. The tumor should be completely excised. If this is not a feasible option then a debulking procedure is performed. Post operative radiotherapy can be used to limit further growth. Options include external beam or stereotactic radiotherapy.

The surgical approach to resection depends on the size and extent of the tumor. An endoscopic nasal approach can be used for tumors limited to the nasopharynx, nasal cavity, and paranasal sinuses. More extensive disease will necessitate an external or a combined approach. A lateral rhinotomy, infratemporal fossa approach, and midfacial degloving are common approaches for larger tumors. Preoperative embolization is performed in hypervascular tumors.

JUVENILE NASAL ANGIOFIBROMAS

These are composed of dense fibrous tissue interlaced with variable amounts of endothelium-lined vascular spaces. They are found exclusively in adolescent boys and arise from mucosa around the sphenopalatine foramen. They present primarily with sinonasal symptoms. They stop growing with age but can become very large and extend into paranasal sinuses, orbit, pterygomaxillary space, and cavernous sinus. Treatment is by surgical excision. Hormonal treatment and radiation therapy have been described (see Fig. 2.2.2A–D in chap. 2.2).

SQUAMOUS PAPILLOMAS

These can be subclassified into inverting, fungiform, and cylindrical depending on their histological appearance. Inverting papillomas involve the nasopharynx and skull base more often than the other types; they originate from the maxillary antrum, ethmoid sinus and lateral nasal wall (Fig. 3.1.3). They have a significant risk of malignant transformation (15%). Squamous

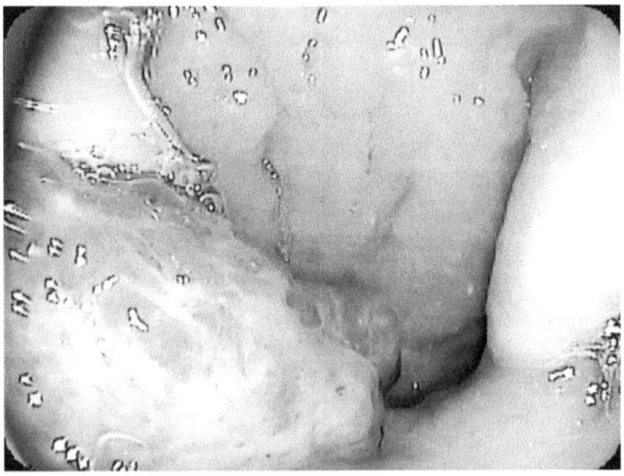

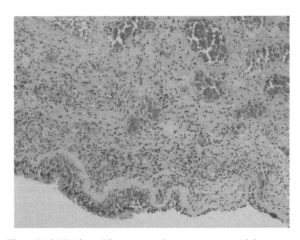

Figure 3.1.1 Hemangioma of right side postnasal space (seen from the left nostril).

Figure 3.1.2 Histology: Edematous respiratory mucosa containing numerous dilated vascular channels consistent with an hemangioma.

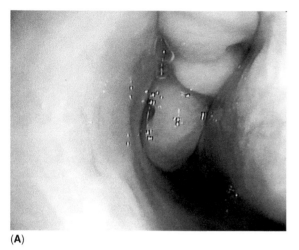

(A)

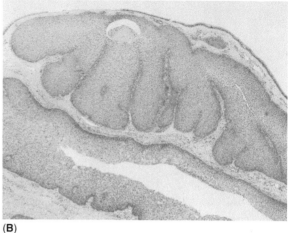

(B)

Figure 3.1.3 (A) Inverted papilloma, left nasal cavity. (B) Histology: A squamous proliferation showing an inverted growth pattern but no dysplasia. The appearance is characteristic of an inverted papilloma.

papilloma can occur at all ages of life, but have a peak incidence between 30 and 50. There is no gender bias. Treatment is by complete resection.

PLEOMORPHIC ADENOMAS

These tumors are exceedingly rare. They arise from nests of minor salivary glands within the nasopharynx as a firm pedunculated mass. They are composed of both epithelial and mesenchymal elements and have a fibrous capsule. Treatment is by surgical resection. Recurrence is high if a significant margin is not obtained.

CEPHALOCELES

Developmental defects in the bony skull base can lead to herniation of intracranial contents. Basal cephaloceles can manifest internally as a nasopharyngeal mass. They are difficult to diagnose as often they present with headache only or if the pituitary stalk is stretched, with hypothalamic pituitary dysfunction. Associated symptoms include visual field defects with the optic tract involvement. They may manifest as chronic nasal discharge or nasal obstruction when endoscopic examination will reveal a mass in the nose. Treatment involves reduction of any herniated brain tissue, resection of any dura with closure of the dural defect, and repair of the bony defect.

RATHKE POUCH

This is an invagination of nasopharyngeal epithelium from which the anterior pituitary gland develops during fetal development. Remnants can persist from which cysts and tumors may form. They rarely cause symptoms and are usually discovered incidentally. Symptoms include post nasal drip, halitosis, Eustachian tube problems, and nasal blockage. The differential diagnosis of a cyst in this location includes Rathke pouch cyst, branchial cleft cyst, Thornwaldt cysts (Fig. 3.1.4), and adenoidal retention cysts. It is also important to consider an

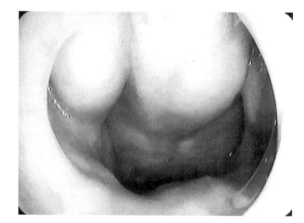

Figure 3.1.4 A Thornwaldt cyst.

encephalocele, meningocele, and a meningomyelocele. They can occur at any age, but have a peak incidence between 50 and 60. They seldom require treatment.

CHORDOMAS

These benign tumors originate from notochord remnants. They can be very aggressive locally and tend to recur after removal. Skull base chordomas most commonly present as a nasopharyngeal mass and tend to present in a younger age group (4th decade) than chordomas elsewhere (6th decade) and have an equal sex distribution again unlike chordomas elsewhere where there is a 2:1 male bias. Complete resection is the treatment of choice.

ADENOIDAL HYPERTROPHY

Adenoids or pharyngeal tonsils are a collection of lymphoid tissue situated in the roof of the nasopharynx. With the palatine,

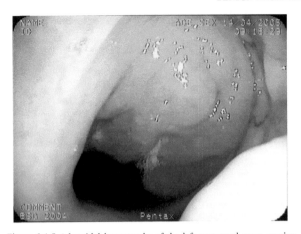

Figure 3.1.5 Adenoidal hypertrophy of the left post nasal space causing obstruction in an adult.

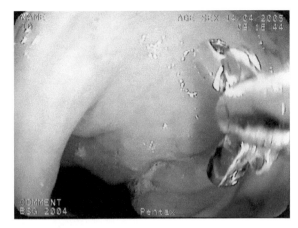

Figure 3.1.6 Biopsy of the adenoidal mass (mentioned in Fig. 3.1.5) in the left post nasal space under local anesthetic in the clinic.

tubal, and lingual tonsils they collectively form Waldeyer's ring and are exposed to antigens from air or food.

While strictly not a tumor, adenoidal hypertrophy is the most commonly seen mass in the nasopharynx (video 6). It is quite normal from the ages of about 6 months to 6 years, when new antigen exposure and development of immune competency is at its highest. They are not infrequently seen in older children as well as adults (Figs. 3.1.5–3.1.7). Excessive adenoid tissue can present in a variety of ways but the symptoms are usually due to infection and inflammation or obstruction.

Acute adenoiditis symptoms include purulent nasal discharge, nasal obstruction, fever, and otalgia due to a secondary acute otitis media. Chronic adenoiditis symptoms include persistent nasal discharge, postnasal drip, and halitosis. Symptoms of obstructive adenoid hyperplasia include chronic nasal obstruction, nasal discharge, snoring, mouth breathing, and a hyponasal voice. In combination with tonsillar hypertrophy it can lead to obstructive sleep apnea, marked by loud snoring, apneic episodes while sleeping, daytime somnolence, behavioral problems, and enuresis.

Medical treatments for adenoid hyperplasia include antibiotic therapy and a prolonged course of nasal steroids. The benefits of such treatment are uncertain, however.

Surgical management involves a complete excision of the offending adenoids. Currently accepted indications for

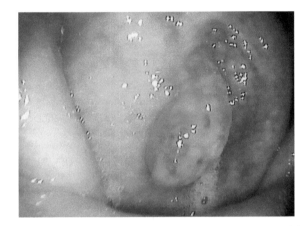

Figure 3.1.7 An unusual polypoid, adenoidal hypertrophy seen in an adult patient.

adenoidectomy include obstructive sleep apnea, cardiopulmonary complications associated with upper airways obstruction, persistent middle ear effusion for more than 3 months, or a second set of ventilation tubes. Other symptoms include a recurrent acute or chronic adenoiditis, recurrent bouts of acute otitis media, hyponasal speech, and orofacial growth disturbance.

3.2.1 Oropharynx tumors
Tom Wilson

The oropharynx is part of the pharynx and is located as the conduit between the oral cavity, nasopharynx, and hypopharynx. The margins are the anterior faucial pillars, the tongue posterior to the circumvallate papillae (tongue base), the valleculae, the inferior mucosal surface of the soft palate, and the posterior pharyngeal wall mucosa between.

PRESENTATION

Benign tumors of the oropharynx represent either epithelial or mesenchymal cellular proliferations.

Epithelial tumors including papillomas, adenomas, and pleomorphic adenomas tend to be located on the tonsils or palate and appear often as well-defined pedunculated masses. Mesenchymal tumors of the oropharynx represent soft/connective tissue masses including fibromas, lipomas, myxomas, osteomas, hemangiomas, lymphangiomas, and neuromas. These can occur anywhere within the oropharynx but often involve the tongue. Hemangiomas are most commonly seen in neonates, and cutaneous lesions are thought to affect 12% of term newborns and 22% of preterm infants. The male to female ratio is 1:3. They may present in the oropharynx.

Lingual thyroid tissue appears as a midline mass in the tongue base with its own unique management issues.

Systemic diseases may manifest themselves as mucosal lesions in the oropharynx. Amyloid of the oropharynx is an extremely rare condition presenting as a smooth mass. Sarcoidosis and pemphigoid may also affect the oropharynx (Figs. 3.2.1.1 & 3.2.1.2).

Mucus retention cysts are common in this area and often referred in the mistaken belief as tumors (Fig. 3.2.1.3).

A final group of benign tumors presenting in the oropharynx are parapharyngeal space masses that displace the lateral oropharyngeal wall. These include benign tumors of the deep lobe of the parotid and vascular tumors and paragangliomas. Tumors present in an insidious manner either as an incidental finding of an asymptomatic smooth swelling during a dental or medical examination, or because the patient is concerned about an asymmetric swelling within the mouth.

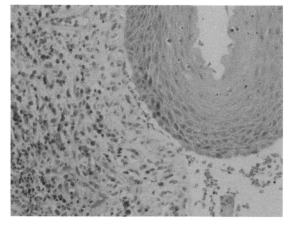

Figure 3.2.1.2 Oral mucosa with subepithelial blister formation, leukocyte exocytosis, and dense mixed inflammation within the subepithelial connective tissue. These are features in keeping with mucous membrane pemphigoid.

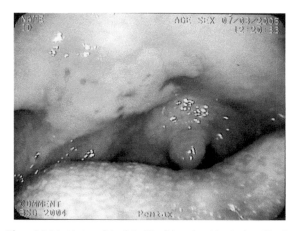

Figure 3.2.1.1 A lesion of the right side of the soft and hard palate. Biopsies proved this to be due to cicatrizing pemphigoid.

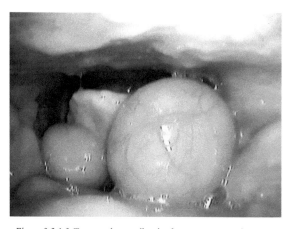

Figure 3.2.1.3 Two very large vallecular fossa mucus retention cysts.

CLINICAL APPEARANCE

Papillomas are associated with human papilloma virus and appear as solitary pedunculated lesions most often on the uvula or free edge of the soft palate or on the tonsil.

Adenomas and pleomorphic adenomas are tumors of the minor salivary glands and present as smooth palatal masses.

Hemangiomas will vary in their appearance from small discrete red macules to massive distorting tumors. They usually appear in the first 3 months after birth followed by a growth phase and then an involution and regression phase that may persist up to 10 years.

Lingual thyroid is a thyroid tissue that has undergone maldescent from its embryological origin in the tongue base (foramen cecum). It enlarges as the child grows. It appears as a midline tongue base mass often causing dysphagia or dysphonia. *Amyloid deposits* appear as elevated, smooth, mucosa-covered firm masses causing symptoms due to their mass effect.

Parapharyngeal space masses appear as diffuse medial displacement of the lateral wall (tonsils) with perhaps a visible or palpable lateral neck component.

IMAGING

Imaging is rarely required for most of the benign oropharyngeal tumors as their diagnosis is clinically suspected and if necessary confirmed by biopsy. Imaging such as CT or MRI may be indicated to delineate anatomical extension of unusual or large benign oropharyngeal tumors (Figs. 3.2.1.4–3.2.1.6). CT or MRI or both are needed for anatomical delineation of parapharyngeal space masses. Radionucleotide scanning may occasionally be indicated for lingual thyroid masses to ascertain whether there is other functional thyroid tissue present in the neck prior to excision of the lingual thyroid tissue. Amyloid is due to extracellular proteinaceous deposits with characteristic microscopic

(green fluorescence under polarized light after Congo red staining) and ultrastructural features. It may be a localized deposit diagnosed on biopsy or a part of systemic amyloidosis with an

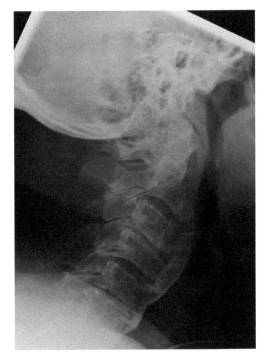

Figure 3.2.1.5 A lateral cervical spine x-ray. Confluent-bridging osteophytes indenting the hypopharynx.

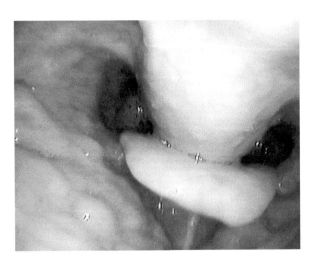

Figure 3.2.1.4 An 80-year-old male with total dysphagia and airway compromise. This large tumor of the posterior pharyngeal wall turned out to be a large anterior cervical osteophyte indenting hypopharynx.

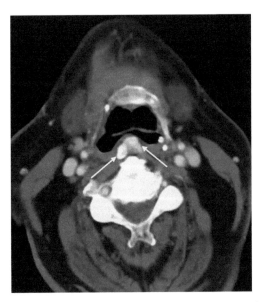

Figure 3.2.1.6 An axial CT scan at the level of the epiglottis. Osteophytes (*arrows*) extending up to the epiglottis.

associated monoclonal lymphoplasmacytic infiltrate. An echo-cardiogram and an ultrasound of the abdomen should be arranged to look for systemic involvement.

MANAGEMENT

The management of benign oropharyngeal tumors requires the confident exclusion of their malignant counterparts. This is sometimes possible on the basis of clinical suspicion and appearance but in many situations will require a biopsy to make the final diagnosis. If the lesion is symptomatic, then the treatment of choice is excision.

Hemangiomas are known to regress spontaneously with a resolution complete by 5 years in about 50% of cases. For this reason aggressive treatment of hemangiomas is seldom indicated. Tumors that compromise the airway or encroach on other vital structures can be treated by high dose corticosteroid therapy, interferon therapy, and very occasionally surgical resection.

Lingual thyroid tissue, if symptomatic, will require excision regardless of whether or not it is the only functioning thyroid tissue.

Papillomas are often solitary pedunculated lesions that have a distinctive clinical appearance and can be safely excised often under local anesthetic. Larger more complex benign lesions with functional compromise may require extensive surgery with reconstruction if necessary although this scenario is rare.

Localized *amyloid* is treated by excision and the systemic variant by chemotherapy.

Parapharyngeal space tumors will be managed by appropriate imaging, a histological diagnosis, and the excision of parapharyngeal mass by either an external or an internal (transtonsillar fossa) approach, taking care to minimize the risk to the neurovascular structures intrinsic to the area.

3.2.2 Benign parapharyngeal tumors affecting the tonsils
Hemi Patel

Parapharyngeal tumors are rare and account for only 0.5% of all head and neck tumors. Eighty percent of these tumors are benign and the vast majority can be classified as either salivary gland neoplasms (50%) or neurogenic tumors (30%).

Clinically, the parapharynx should be considered as two spaces divided by the styloid apparatus into pre- and post-styloid compartments. The pre-styloid space contains the deep lobe of the parotid gland, minor salivary glands, and fat. The post-styloid compartment contains the internal carotid artery, internal jugular vein, cranial nerves IX to XII, cervical sympathetic chain, and lymph nodes.

SALIVARY GLAND NEOPLASMS
These arise from the pre-styloid space, from the deep lobe of the parotid or minor salivary gland tissue and account for 50% of parapharyngeal space (PPS) lesions.

Ninety percent of these are pleomorphic adenomas (Figs. 3.2.2.1–3.2.2.3). Others include Warthin's tumors and oncocytomas.

NEUROGENIC NEOPLASMS
Neurogenic tumors are the second most common PPS tumor and represent 30% of the cases. They arise from the post-styloid compartment.

Schwannomas
Schwannomas account for the majority of Neurogenic tumors, arising most commonly from the vagus nerve (50%) or the

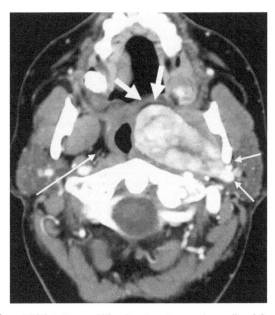

Figure 3.2.2.2 A 60-year-old female patient. Symptomless swelling, left oropharynx and soft palate. Pleomorphic adenoma arising from the deep lobe of the left parotid gland. Axial CT scan post contrast. Enhancing mass effacing the left parapharyngeal fat and indenting the left oropharynx. The lesion arises exophytically from the deep lobe of parotid (*short arrows*). Note the anteromedial displacement of the parapharyngeal fat (*thick white arrows*). Normal right parapharyngeal fat (*long arrow*).

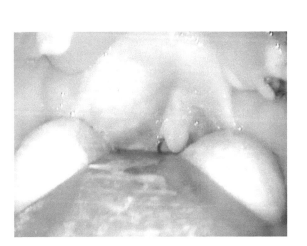

Figure 3.2.2.1 Parapharyngeal pleomorphic adenoma pushing the soft palate and tonsil down and forward on right side.

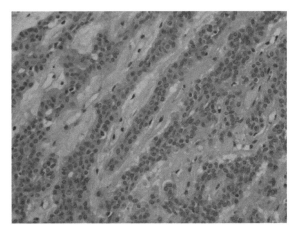

Figure 3.2.2.3 An encapsulated tumor composed predominantly of trabeculae of myoepithelial cells in a myxoid stroma. The features are those of a pleomorphic adenoma.

sympathetic chain. They are slow growing, encapsulated, and distinct from the nerve of origin. Treatment is by enucleation with sparing of the nerve.

Paragangliomas

These are the second most common neurogenic tumors. They are benign vascular neoplasms that arise from neural crest tissue.

They are associated with the carotid body, jugular bulb, and the vagus nerve and are called carotid body tumors, glomus jugulare, and glomus vagale respectively (Figs. 3.2.2.4–3.2.2.6).

Neurofibromas

Neurofibromas are unencapsulated tumors intimately related to the nerve from which they arise. There can be multiple

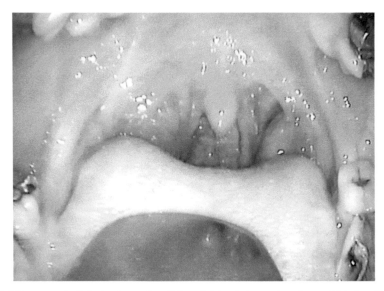

Figure 3.2.2.4 Right sided Glomus vagale displacing the tonsil medially and giving the impression of a very full (enlarged) tonsillar fossa as a result.

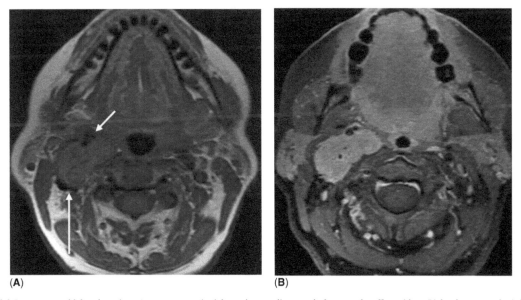

(A) **(B)**

Figure 3.2.2.5 A 50-year-old female patient. An asymptomatic right neck mass discovered after a road traffic accident. Right glomus vagale. (A) Axial T1 image. Intermediate signal mass splaying the internal jugular vein (*long arrow*) and the carotid arteries (*short arrow*) just above the carotid bifurcation. Lesion located in the carotid space. (B) Axial T1 fatsat image post gadolinium. Lesion enhances vividly and almost uniformly.

neurofibromas and they are associated with neurofibromatosis. In contrast to schwannomas they paralyze the associated nerve, have a small risk of undergoing malignant transformation, and are usually excised sacrificing the associated nerve.

PRESENTATION

Clinical detection of a parapharyngeal tumor is often difficult and the presentation very subtle. They usually present as an asymptomatic mass causing mild bulging of the soft palate, tonsillar fossa, or fullness at the angle of the mandible. Tumors must be at least 2 cm before they become clinically apparent and often they are discovered incidentally.

Medial extension of the tumor can cause unilateral Eustachian tube dysfunction associated with middle ear effusion and

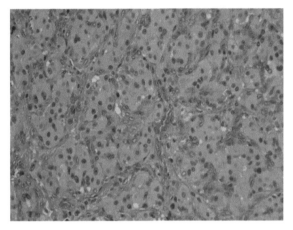

Figure 3.2.2.6 Paraganglioma. Histology: The tumor has an organoid "zell-ballen" architecture and is composed of cells with round to oval nuclei and abundant eosinophilic cytoplasm. Between the cells are spindled or sustentacular cells.

hearing loss. Distortion of the oropharynx can cause dysphagia, dyspnea, and obstructive sleep apnea.

Post-styloid lesions can cause compression of cranial nerves IX–XII and therefore cause hoarseness of voice, dysphagia, dysarthria, and a Horner's syndrome.

Parapharyngeal tumors may mimic a peritonsillar abscess and cause delay in diagnosis.

IMAGING

Radiology is vital in the assessment of PPS masses. A presumptive diagnosis can be made in most cases on imaging, often negating the need for a needle or open biopsy.

CT, MRI, and angiography can all be useful in evaluating the tumor.

CT scan will show a parotid tumor in the pre-styloid space displacing the carotid posteriorly. Neurogenic tumors are usually found in the post-styloid space and push the carotid anteriorly. They appear characteristically enhanced on CT.

MRI provides more accurate information on the extent of the tumor and its relations to surround soft tissue structures, especially the carotid artery.

If a carotid involvement is suspected, an angiogram will define the vascular anatomy and enable possible preoperative embolization.

MANAGEMENT

With a 10-year survival for benign parapharyngeal tumors approaching the 100% mark, a careful consideration of tumor behavior, risk of neurovascular complications, patient age, and fitness is crucial. Surgery is the mainstay of treatment, but simple observation, or external beam or stereotactic radiotherapy should be considered in elderly and surgically unfit patients.

The two main surgical approaches are transcervical for post-styloid tumors and transparotid for pre-styloid tumors. Often a combined approach can be utilized with a mandibulotomy to increase exposure.

3.3.1 Supraglottis
Mike Thomas

AMYLOID

This is a rare laryngeal condition accounting for less than 1% of all benign laryngeal tumors. Localized amyloidosis is characterized by the deposition of amyloid fibers within the larynx in the absence of systemic involvement. It can affect all three subdivisions of the larynx. It can present with long-standing hoarseness or dyspnea. Diagnosis is by clinical suspicion and CT scanning, and a two-dimensional reconstruction may help localize the lesion and plan surgery. Staining with Congo red and examination with polarized light microscopy will confirm the diagnosis. An endoscopic excision should give excellent results but repeated removals may be necessary (Figs. 3.3.1.1–3.3.1.3).

ONCOCYTIC CYSTS/ONCOCYTOMAS

These are rare, benign and slow-growing cystic lesions arising in the minor salivary glands. They occur in the ventricles of the false vocal folds due to oncocytic metaplasia in the laryngeal epithelium. Usually, these occur in the elderly and are usually solitary. Symptoms include hoarseness, pain, and stridor. The term "prolapse of the ventricle" has been used to describe their appearance in the supraglottic larynx. Treatment is by local endoscopic excision, but recurrences cannot be avoided (Figs. 3.3.1.4 & 3.3.1.5).

SACCULAR CYSTS

Several types of laryngeal cysts have been described with various classifications depending on the anatomical sites and pathological findings. Saccular cysts are uncommon disorders that represent cystic dilatation of the laryngeal saccule; unlike laryngoceles they do not contain air. In adults voice change is a common symptom, but they can distort the airway if large in size and an airway compromise can occur, especially in infants. CT scanning will demonstrate the extent of the cyst. MRI scanning may demonstrate a rounded nonenhancing mass. Tracheostomy may be needed in the pediatric population but the preferred treatment is an endoscopic removal. An external approach may be needed in adults.

LARYNGOCELES

Laryngoceles develop within the saccule of the laryngeal ventricle (video 10); they are rare, more common in men, usually developing in the 6th decade. The majority are unilateral (Figs. 3.3.1.6–3.3.1.8). They are divided into external (30%), internal (20%), and combined (50%) tumors. They usually present with hoarseness or a neck swelling. Rarely, they can give rise to stridor or a sore throat; they can become infected. Treatment is between surgical excision by an external approach and endoscopic laser marsupialization. Rarely, they can contain a carcinoma.

NEUROENDOCRINE TUMORS

Neuroendocrine tumors can basically be divided into two main subclasses: those that arise from neural tissue (paragangliomas) and are generally benign and those arising from the epithelial cells (carcinoid, atypical carcinoid, and small cell carcinomata).

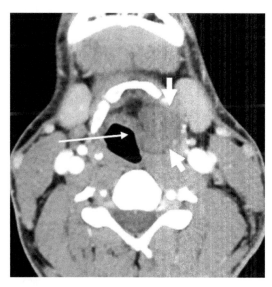

Figure 3.3.1.2 Supraglottic amyloid. Axial postcontrast CT images of the supraglottic larynx at the level of hyoid. Soft tissue attenuation mass (*thick arrows*) displacing the epiglottis (*arrow*) to the right, and extending into the pre-epiglottic fat.

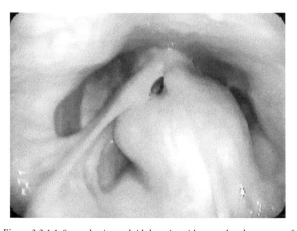

Figure 3.3.1.1 Supraglottic amyloid deposits with smooth enlargement of the left aryepiglottic fold and false cord with the glottis completely obscured.

Paragangliomas of the larynx are rare and arise from the paired laryngeal paraganglion cells located in the false vocal folds in association with the internal branch of the superior laryngeal nerve. They also arise from the posterior branch of the recurrent laryngeal nerve and can give rise to a subglottic swelling. They occur most frequently in the supraglottis (82%), presenting with hoarseness and dysphagia and clinically look like a submucosal mass; they often have an extensive vascular makeup. They are rarely functional and seldom associated with other paragangliomas. They are more common in women than men and the ratio is 3:1, presenting usually between 50 and 70 years of age. Conservative surgical removal is the treatment of choice and the overall prognosis is excellent.

SCHWANNOMAS

These are uncommon nerve sheath tumors that usually occur within the aryepiglottic folds associated with the internal branch of the superior laryngeal nerve. They are more common in women, usually occurring between the ages of 40 and 50, having an insidious course. Tumors are usually small and solitary,

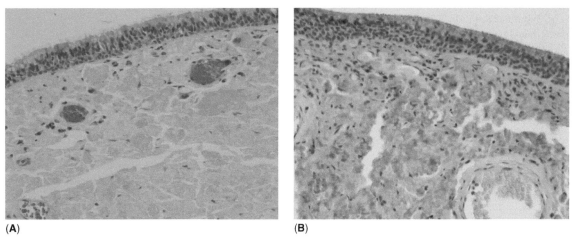

(A) (B)

Figure 3.3.1.3 (**A**) and (**B**) Laryngeal mucosa containing amorphous pink material in the subepithelial connective tissue. This stains "brick red" on Congo red stain, consistent with amyloid deposition.

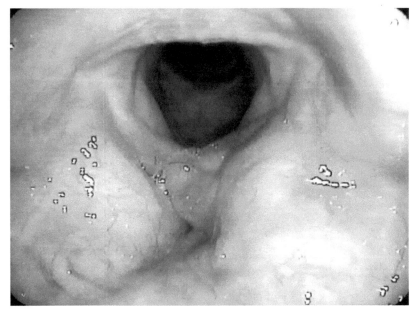

Figure 3.3.1.4 An oncocytic metaplastic benign minor salivary gland cyst distorting the supraglottis and obscuring the view of the anterior vocal cords.

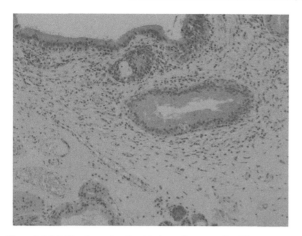

Figure 3.3.1.5 Histology: A polypoid piece of mucosa, lined by squamous and respiratory epithelium, containing salivary gland tissue which shows an oncocytic change and mucin-filled cyst formation.

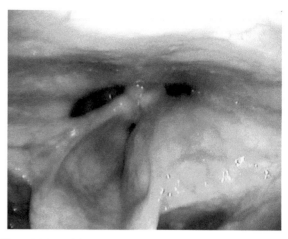

Figure 3.3.1.8 A left-sided unilateral laryngocele with expansion of the pharyngoepiglottic fold.

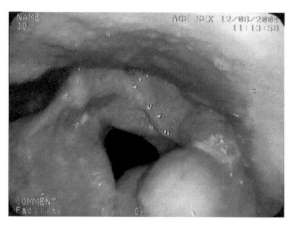

Figure 3.3.1.6 Bilateral internal laryngoceles. Left side larger than the right. Photograph taken when laryngoceles "deflated" at rest.

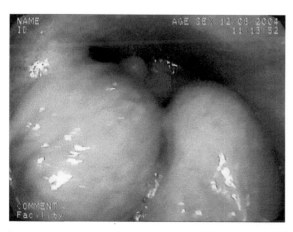

Figure 3.3.1.7 Laryngoceles fully inflated on vocalizing, obstructing the view of the larynx.

causing a localized swelling, or an area of inflammation or ulceration. Unlike neurofibromas, they are well encapsulated and the nerve lies stretched over the surface of the tumor. They can be treated by endoscopic removal.

NEUROFIBROMAS

Laryngeal neurofibromas may be solitary and nonsyndromic, or more commonly multiple and associated with neurofibromatosis type 1 or 2. They are rare and generally involve the aryepiglottic folds and the arytenoids. The tumors arising from the superior laryngeal nerve itself or the anastomosis with the recurrent laryngeal nerve. Symptoms include progressive stridor, hoarseness, and dysphagia. Neurofibromas can be symptom free for years due to their location and slow growth. They appear as a pink/yellow submucosal mass with prominent vascularity along the aryepiglottic fold. Histologically there is a diffuse fusiform swelling consisting of both neural and fibrous tissues; the nerve is encased within the tumor. Imaging would involve either a contrast-enhanced CT scan or an MRI scan. Sagittal images are useful. There is no consensus on the best approach to treatment; it may range from endoscopic removal of small localized lesions, to conservative surgery to preserve laryngeal function. Recurrence or residual disease can be dealt with by endoscopic laser excision.

LIPOMAS

Usually occur in the supraglottic larynx as a fatty deposit within the false vocal folds. They can present at all ages and if symptomatic can be removed surgically.

OTHER TUMORS

Tumors may arise from all tissue layers in the supraglottis. Tumors arising from the muscle layers are rarely seen (Figs. 3.3.1.9–3.3.1.11). Those arising from the blood vessels (hemangiomas)

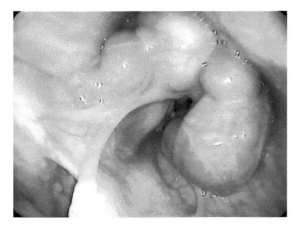

Figure 3.3.1.9 Benign rhabdomyoma arising from the striated muscle of the supraglottis.

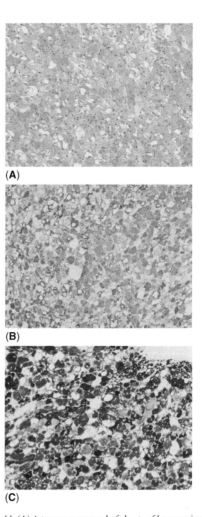

(A)

(B)

(C)

Figure 3.3.1.11 (A) A tumor composed of sheets of large eosinophilic cells with granular, vacuolated cytoplasm and small nuclei. The cells show diffuse cytoplasmic staining with myoglobin (B) and desmin (C). The features are those of an adult rhabdomyoma.

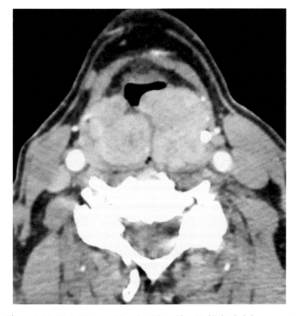

Figure 3.3.1.10 A 67-year-old male with stridor. Multiple rhabdomyomata of the supraglottic larynx. An axial CT post contrast through the larynx. Section at the level of the thyrohyoid membrane showing large bilateral masses with a compromise of the supraglottic airway.

are more commonly seen (Fig. 3.3.1.12). Mucus retention cysts arise in minor salivary glands as a result of blockage of the glandular outflow (Fig. 3.3.1.13).

Systemic diseases such as sarcoidosis and cicatricial pemphigoid can also affect the supraglottis as can infective diseases such as viral papillomas (Figs. 3.3.1.14–3.3.1.18).

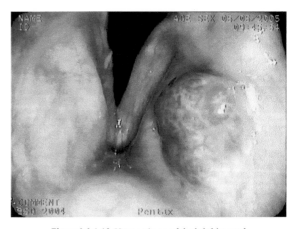

Figure 3.3.1.12 Hemangioma of the left false cord.

69

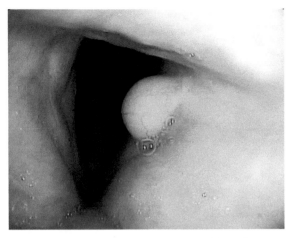

Figure 3.3.1.13 Mucus retention cyst, left false cord.

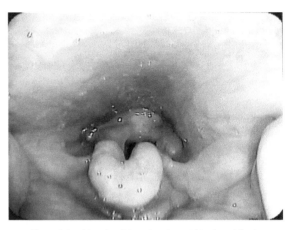

Figure 3.3.1.16 Isolated deposits of sarcoid in the epiglottis.

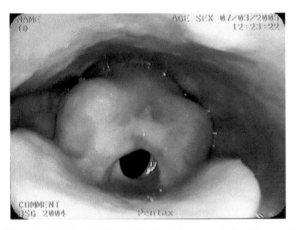

Figure 3.3.1.14 Cicatricial pemphigoid of the supraglottis with normal glottis beneath the affected tissue.

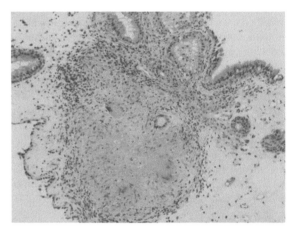

Figure 3.3.1.17 Histology: Respiratory epithelium containing well-defined "naked" granulomas and scattered giant cells in keeping with sarcoidosis.

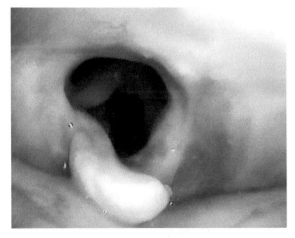

Figure 3.3.1.15 Sarcoid deposits and deformity of the epiglottis, aryepi-glottic folds, and inter-arytenoid area.

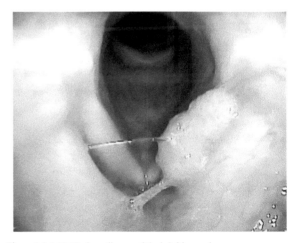

Figure 3.3.1.18 Viral papillomas of the left false cord.

3.3.2 Glottis
Mike Thomas

HYPERKERATOSIS

This appears as a white thickening over part or the entire vocal fold; it may be unilateral or bilateral. It is due to excess protein deposition within the superficial layers of the vocal fold. There is usually a history of chronic irritation that can include voice overuse, smoking, and asthma with steroid inhalation. The differential diagnosis would include dysplasia and carcinoma *in situ*. Histological assessment using microlaryngeal techniques is needed to obtain a biopsy (Fig. 3.3.2.1).

PAPILLOMATOSIS

It is the most common of all the benign laryngeal tumors, usually located on the vocal folds but can involve the trachea and lower respiratory tract. Can occur at all ages and are broadly divided into adult papillomatosis (25%) where the lesions are usually single and juvenile papillomatosis (85%) with multiple lesions. They are caused by the human papilloma virus types 6 and 11. Hoarseness is a common symptom but stridor can occur with extensive multiple lesions. Clinically the lesions can be soft or firm with frond-like projections arising from the vocal folds; some lesions have a broad base. Recurrence is common but malignant transformation is rare. Various treatments have been attempted, new antivirals have been tested, and surgical removal using laser and laryngeal debriders has been used, but often in children multiple procedures are required (Figs. 3.3.2.2–3.3.2.4).

POLYPS

Vocal fold polyps are unilateral and usually involve the free edge of the true vocal fold but can also arise from the superior or inferior borders. These are more common in men and are usually caused by intense vocal abuse. They can be sessile with a broad based or pedunculated having a small stalk (Figs. 3.3.2.5–3.3.2.7). Microlaryngoscopy with careful biopsy is usually needed followed by voice therapy. Rhabdomyoma can present as a polypoid mass affecting the vocal folds, and the conservative surgical excision is the treatment of choice.

NODULES

Vocal fold nodules are localized, benign, superficial growths that occur on the medial aspect on the anterior two-thirds of the vocal folds. They are usually bilateral and classically arise from the junction of the anterior and middle third of the true

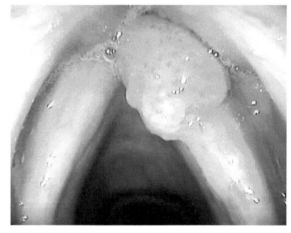
Figure 3.3.2.2 Respiratory papillomas arising from the anterior third of the right vocal cord and anterior commissure.

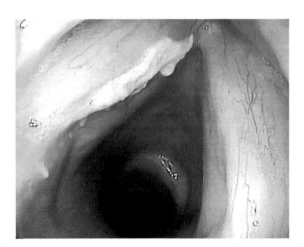
Figure 3.3.2.1 Hyperkeratosis of the left vocal cord.

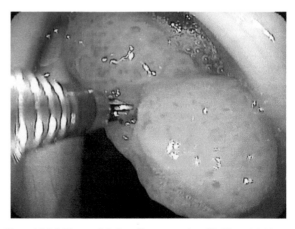
Figure 3.3.2.3 Biopsy of viral papillomas mentioned in Figure 3.3.2.2.

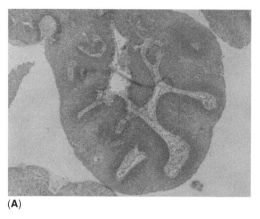
(A)

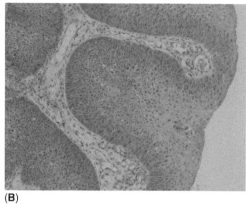
(B)

Figure 3.3.2.4 Histology: (**A**) Laryngeal mucosa showing a florid epithelial proliferation and low grade dysplasia at high power (**B**), consistent with a squamous papilloma.

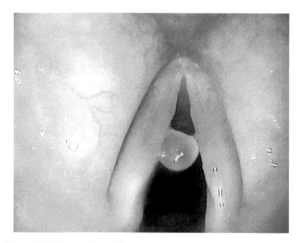

Figure 3.3.2.5 A cystic-type laryngeal polyp arising from the leading edge of the left vocal cord.

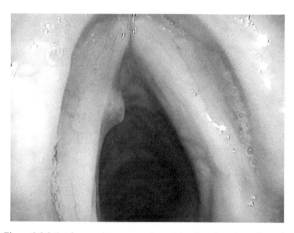

Figure 3.3.2.6 A hemangiomatous polyp arising from junction of anterior and middle third of left vocal cord.

vocal fold (Figs. 3.3.2.8 & 3.3.2.9). These probably develop as a result of phonotrauma; they are seen more frequently in women aged 20–50 years. They also occur in children and are commonly called "screamer" nodules. Symptoms include hoarseness, voice breaks, and vocal fatigue. Diagnosis is aided by flexible endoscopy and stroboscope. Treatment is by reassurance, vocal hygiene, and speech therapy.

REINKE'S EDEMA
This condition is a diffuse polypoid degeneration that occurs in Reinke's space. It is usually bilateral giving rise to a deep husky voice. The condition maintains an eponymous title being named after Friedrich Berthold Reinke, a German anatomist who described the condition in 1895. It is more common in women as is associated with voice misuse, smoking, and hypothyroidism. Clinically the appearance is that of a gelatinous swelling beneath the vocal fold mucosa. Treatment involves

speech therapy and removal of the swelling by microsurgical techniques (Fig. 3.3.2.10).

CYSTS
Laryngeal cysts are rare benign lesions that can affect all age groups, especially singers. Two types are usually found occurring within Reinke's space, *mucus retention cysts* and *epidermoid cysts* that can contain epithelium or accumulated keratin. Mucus retention cysts occur spontaneously while epidermoid cysts are associated with vocal abuse. Symptoms include hoarseness, vocal fatigue, and soreness. Management is a combination of speech therapy and microsurgical excision.

GRANULOMAS
Granulomas are benign lesions usually located on the posterior third of the vocal fold adjacent to the vocal process of the arytenoids. They can be unilateral or bilateral. They are more

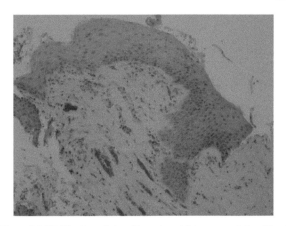

Figure 3.3.2.7 Histology: Polypoid vocal cord biopsy containing dilated capillaries consistent with a hemangiomatous polyp (H&E x100).

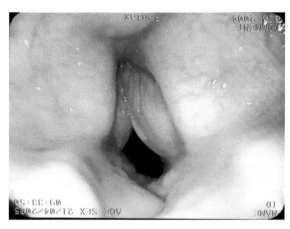

Figure 3.3.2.10 Reinke's edema affecting the right vocal cord more than the left.

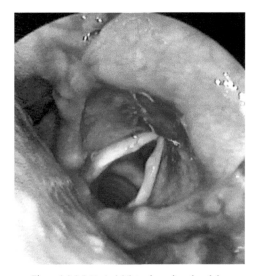

Figure 3.3.2.8 Typical, bilateral vocal cord nodules.

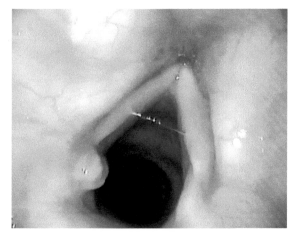

Figure 3.3.2.11 A typical granuloma arising from the left vocal process.

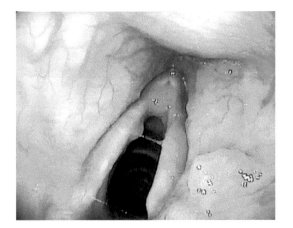

Figure 3.3.2.9 A unilateral vocal nodule. There is also a small papilloma in the anterior commissure.

common in men and have a range of etiological factors from voice abuse, trauma from intubation to laryngopharyngeal reflux disease. The underlying cause needs to be treated but the lesions are usually biopsied to get a definitive diagnosis; they can be very resistant to treatment (Fig. 3.3.2.11).

GRANULAR CELL TUMORS

These can arise within the vocal folds and present with hoarseness. There is no specific age incidence. They appear as a small, firm sessile lesion with an intact mucosa. They are thought to arise from undifferentiated mesenchymal or Schwann cells. Treatment is by endoscopic surgical removal.

3.3.3   Subglottis
Mike Thomas

CYSTS

Subglottic cysts are rare and are usually associated with endotracheal intubation in preterm infants. They are removed endoscopically but there can be recurrences.

CHONDROMAS

These are slow-growing cartilaginous tumors. Seventy percent of all laryngeal chondromas arise from the posterior cricoid plate. There is a 5 to 1 incidence in men and women, usually occurring between 40 and 60 years of age. They appear as a smooth encapsulated tumor with an intact mucosa. Radiologically they can display mottled calcification. Surgical excision with or without cricoid reconstruction is advised.

ADENOMAS

These are benign tumors that arise from seromucinous glands within the subglottis. They are rare and present with stridor; the overlying mucosa is smooth and they need to be distinguished from an adenoid cystic carcinoma.

HEMANGIOMAS

Small cavernous hemangiomas can arise in any part of the larynx but more frequently in the subglottis. These can be removed endoscopically. Capillary hemangiomas are congenital, usually presenting in infants less than 6 months of age. These are not true tumors and usually regress spontaneously.

GRANULOMAS

Granulation tissue may present in the subglottis and upper trachea as a complication of endotracheal intubation or tracheostomy (Fig. 3.3.3.1).

SYSTEMIC DISEASES

Systemic diseases such as Wegener's granulomatosis and pemphigoid may present with lesions in the subglottis and upper trachea (Figs. 3.3.3.2–3.3.3.5).

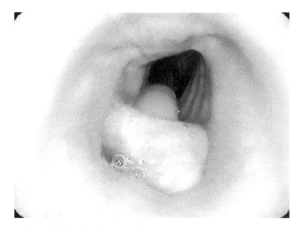

Figure 3.3.3.1 Florid granulation tissue above a tracheostomy tube.

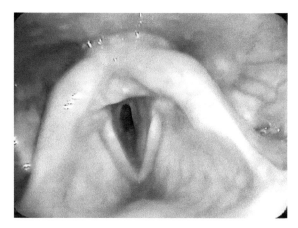

Figure 3.3.3.2 Subglottic stenosis due to Wegener's granulomatosis.

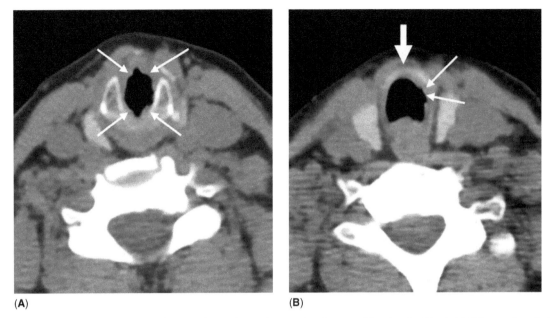

(A)   **(B)**

Figure 3.3.3.3 A 64-year-old female patient with Wegener's granulomatosis. Increasing shortness of breath and stridor. Axial CT images through the subglottic region. (A) Level of posterior cricoid cartilage. An irregular soft tissue thickening (*arrows*) in the subglottis immediately below the vocal cords. (B) Level of the anterior cricoid ring (*thick arrow*). Discrete ulceration (*arrows*) in the left lateral wall.

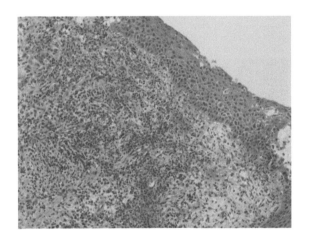

Figure 3.3.3.4 Histology: Inflamed mucosa showing collections of histiocytes within the subepithelial connective tissue, focal necrosis, and early vasculitis in keeping with Wegener's granulomatosis.

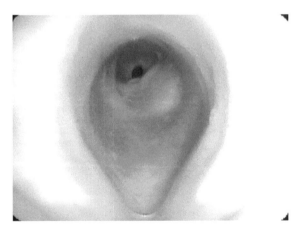

Figure 3.3.3.5 An upper tracheal stenosis due to pemphigoid seen from the level of the vocal cords.

4.1 Endolaryngeal laser surgery using TNLE
Tim Price

INTRODUCTION

Some patients are difficult or impossible to perform rigid laryngoscopy on, for anatomical reasons. In others, it would be hazardous to attempt to administer a general anesthetic because of severe medical comorbidities. In these circumstances the ENT surgeon is faced with a challenge if the patient has pathology of the larynx, which requires a biopsy for tissue diagnosis and possibly further surgical management. TNLE is particularly useful in these circumstances (video 11).

This chapter gives a detailed description of the use of the Nd:YAG laser (wavelength 1064 nm) to obliterate a vocal cord papilloma that could not be visualized by rigid endoscopy.

PROCEDURE

The technique was carried out in the operating theater so that proper laser safety protocols were followed. The endoscope was passed in the usual manner and the vocal cords were anesthetized as described in chapter 1.2 (Fig. 4.1.1). A Pentax Biopsy Forceps (KW1811S) (Slough, U.K.) was passed down the instrument channel to obtain a tissue sample for histology as described in chapter 1.1 and 1.2.

The TNLE was then removed and a 0.6-mm glass optical fiber was passed down the instrument channel and the end was cleaved, ready for use. The fiber was then withdrawn until it was just protruding from the end of the scope and the TNLE scope was then reintroduced via the nose.

The Nd:YAG laser was used because it would not destroy the distally positioned camera chip as a potassium-titanyl-phosphate (or KTP) laser would. The laser was used in the contact mode on a setting of 30 watts at 0.5-second bursts. The authors found out that the most effective way to deal with a large lesion was to target the base of the lesion (Fig. 4.1.2). For smaller lesions, the laser was passed over the surface of the lesion (Fig. 4.1.3). Any smoke produced by the laser was suctioned away using the suction port of the endoscope which was attached to the traditional laser suction device.

As a precaution, the patient was observed overnight before discharge. Three doses of intravenous steroids where given in order to prevent any excessive laryngeal swelling postoperatively. The above settings were effective and appeared to be safe as the patient did not experience any complications or discomfort during the procedure and his voice quality postoperatively was good with complete resolution of the lesions at 6 weeks (Fig. 4.1.4).

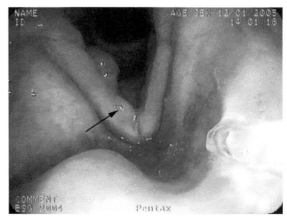

Figure 4.1.1 The large and small (*arrowed*) papillomas are evident and the epidural catheter is in place with a local anesthetic being dripped onto the laryngeal mucosa.

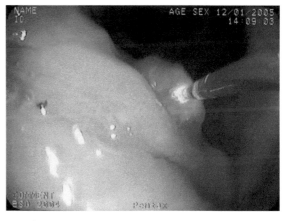

Figure 4.1.2 Laser being used on the larger vocal cord lesion.

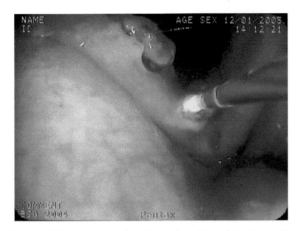

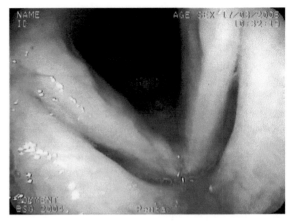

Figure 4.1.3 Laser being used on the surface of the smaller lesion. The larger lesion has been ablated at the base.

Figure 4.1.4 Six weeks postoperatively there is no sign of the lesions.   *Source:* Price T, Sharma A, Montgomery P. "How we do it: vocal cord Nd:Yag laser surgery, under local anaesthetic using a transnasal flexible laryngo-oesophagoscope (TNLE)." Published online in Lasers In Medical Science, January 2007.

2.8 Tracheal tumors
Wyn Parry

PRESENTATION
Although this may be with immediate and catastrophic airway obstruction, this is unusual and the more usual presentation is with insidious and progressive dyspnea. Cough, hemoptysis, and stridor may develop though the latter is unusual as an early feature. Increasing dyspnea, sometimes accompanied by wheeze, leads to asthma or emphysema being erroneously diagnosed, and frequently patients have symptoms for many (typically 6–10) months before a tracheal tumor is diagnosed. Recurrent laryngeal nerve paralysis may be a presentation, but is uncommon.

EPIDEMIOLOGY
Primary malignant tracheal tumors are relatively unusual, with an overall incidence of 0.1 per 100,000. Most will be adenoid cystic or squamous cell carcinomas, the former more common than the latter. The male: female incidence is 2:1 overall and smoking is the commonest recognized etiological factor for squamous cell types, where most patients will be in the 50–70 year age group. Adenoid cystic carcinomas (arising from the bronchial glands) are less predictably related to smoking and these tend to occur across a wider age range 20–80 and with minimal male:female differences in incidence.

Forty percent of patients with a primary tracheal tumor will have prior, concurrent, or subsequent malignancies in the upper aero-digestive tract or lung.

Other primary tracheal malignancies are much rarer still, including carcinoid and other neuroendocrine tumors.

Tracheal invasion by malignancies in related structures (thyroid, esophagus, and lymph nodes) may occur, though a true metastatic disease is rare in the trachea (Figs. 2.8.1–2.8.7).

Benign tracheal tumors are also uncommon and include squamous papilloma, typical carcinoid, and cartilaginous tumors.

HISTOLOGY AND CLINICAL APPEARANCE
The histological appearances of primary tracheal squamous cell carcinoma and carcinoid (typical and atypical) are little different from their counterparts in the lung and elsewhere. Adenoid

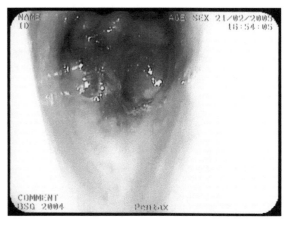

Figure 2.8.2 Endoscope passed through the cords in order to biopsy the tumor.

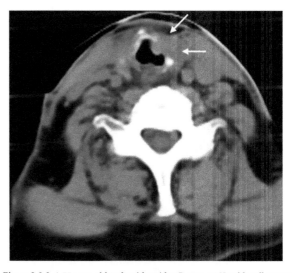

Figure 2.8.3 A 75-year-old male with stridor. Recurrent Hurthle cell tumor of the thyroid invading the trachea (post thyroidectomy). Axial noncontrast CT scan just below cricoid cartilage. Left paratracheal soft tissue thickening (*arrows*) invading the left lateral wall of the trachea.

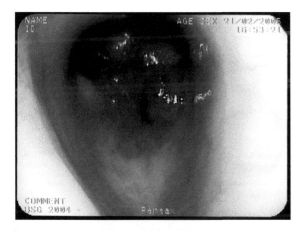

Figure 2.8.1 View of thyroid carcinoma (Hurtle cell) invading the trachea from the level of the vocal cords.

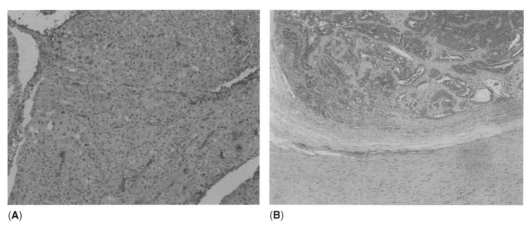

(A)   **(B)**

Figure 2.8.4 (A) A malignant neoplasm composed of large pleomorphic cells with round to oval nuclei, containing prominent nucleoli, and with abundant eosinophilic cytoplasm. (B) Capsular invasion is present. The appearance is that of a Hurthle cell carcinoma.

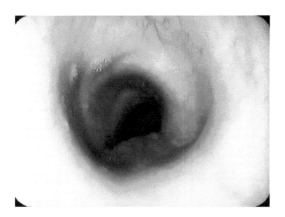

Figure 2.8.5 Post cricoid tumor invading the trachea.

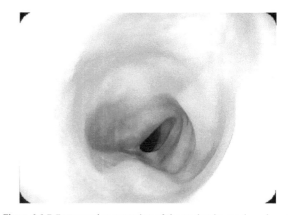

Figure 2.8.7 Extramural compression of the trachea by esophageal carcinoma.

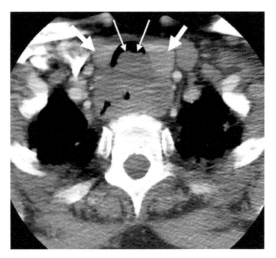

Figure 2.8.6 A 74-year-old female with stridor and dysphagia. Post cricoid carcinoma invading the trachea. Axial post contrast image at and just below the level of the thyroid gland (*thick arrows*) showing a large eccentric post cricoid squamous cell carcinoma invading the trachea (*arrows*).

cystic carcinoma is often slow growing in many patients even after metastases have occurred to extra-tracheal sites. Submucosal and lymphatic spreads are typical with adenoid cystic tumors, often extending for some distance away from an obvious macroscopic tumor and leading to both circumferential and longitudinal spread.

Most tracheal tumors will present at TNLE or bronchoscopy as exophytic masses within the tracheal lumen. Squamous carcinomas frequently ulcerate and metastasize, leading to palpable cervical lymphadenopathy. Adenoid cystic carcinomas frequently present as a rounded mass and the tracheal mucosa may appear normal, with much of the tumor being more submucosally located and a regional lymph node involvement being much less common.

IMAGING

Chest x-ray is often normal, though may show tracheal narrowing, mediastinal widening (both of which can be subtle and easily missed), or occasionally evidence of pulmonary metastases.

CT scanning is useful in visualizing the tracheal mass and assessing the extra-tracheal extent, though it is less accurate in assessing the tumor length. Invasion of surrounding structures can be difficult to assess and though CT may be of use, MRI may be more suitable. PET scanning, particularly in the assessment of potential metastatic sites, also has a role (Figs. 2.8.3, 2.8.6, 2.8.8 & 2.8.9).

Rigid bronchoscopic inspection is essential for complete assessment and treatment planning, both in terms of obtaining tissue for diagnosis and also for assessing the tumor length and its relation to the subglottis and carina, depending on the precise location of the tumor.

Laryngoscopy is also essential with proximal tumors, in order to assess vocal cord function and subglottic airway involvement.

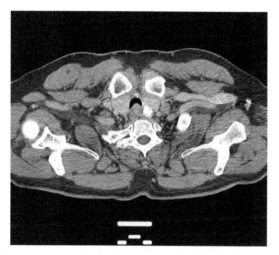

Figure 2.8.8 Cross-sectional imaging of a tracheal tumor arising from the posterior wall of the trachea and indenting the lumen and reducing the airway significantly.

STAGING

There is no specific staging system for tracheal tumors.

MANAGEMENT

Although the optimal management option is tracheal resection, delays in diagnosis are common and many patients will present with inoperable disease due to either local extensions or metastases.

When resection is possible, up to half of the tracheal length can be excised and a primary anastomosis achieved, often without the requirement for any "release" procedures involving either the larynx or the pulmonary hila.

Proximal (subglottic) or distal (carinal) tumors present specific challenges, the former due to the potential requirement for resection of the distal cricoid and laryngeal preservation and the latter due to carinal resection and bronchial re-implantation.

Frozen section analysis of resection margins, especially with adenoid cystic carcinoma (see the section "Histology" above) is important to attempt clear resection margins, though the impact of this on overall survival is not convincing.

Radiotherapy may be helpful as an alternative to resection in unfit patients with squamous cell carcinomas.

For many patients, palliative interventions will be necessary (and may indeed be the only option) on the basis of the disease extent, tumor location, local invasion, or metastatic disease, or else in patients too unfit to undergo extensive, complex tracheal resections.

Palliative options include Nd:YAG laser, rigid bronchoscopic "de-bulking" and/or the implantation of airway stents. The latter are particularly effective, both solid silicone and covered self-expanding metallic stents.

Survival after resection can be satisfactory, particularly with adenoid cystic carcinomas and five-year survival figures in this group is of the order of 70%. Squamous cell carcinomas are associated with a much poorer outlook and five-year survival of 15–20%.

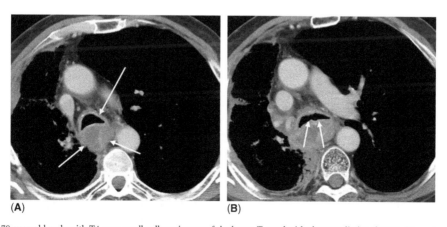

Figure 2.8.9 A 70-year-old male with T4 non–small-cell carcinoma of the lungs. Treated with chemoradiation therapy. Increasing cough and hemoptysis. Axial post contrast CT scans through the carina. (**A**) Soft tissue attenuation mass (*short arrows*) posterior to the carina (*long arrow*). (**B**) Invasion of the posterior carina (*arrows*).

4.2 Direct phonoplasty
Alok Sharma

INTRODUCTION
In patients with unilateral vocal cord palsy, medialization of the paralyzed vocal cord is often used to improve the voice. The concept of the treatment is to medialize the paralyzed vocal cord, facilitating its apposition with the mobile cord during phonation, and thus improving the voice.

There are two established techniques of vocal cord medialization by an injection method. It may be performed with direct laryngoscopy under a general anesthetic, or via a transcricothyroid membrane injection, under a local anesthetic. Both techniques have their advantages and disadvantages.

Direct visualization of the vocal cords, via an operative laryngoscope under a general anesthetic, gives a good visualization of the area to be injected. The surgeon looks directly at the vocal cords and is able to inject into the superior surface of the cords. The principal disadvantage of this technique is that the surgeon can only estimate the amount of injected material to be delivered as the patient is unconscious and therefore unable to phonate (there is no patient feedback). Technically, it may be impossible due to lack of cervical spine extension, or anatomically, the anesthetic tube may obstruct adequate visualization of the vocal cords. Furthermore, the patient may not be fit for a general anesthetic due to coexisting pathology.

The second method is transcricothyroid injection of the vocal cords, under local anesthetic in an outpatient or a day-case setting. A simple flexible nasolaryngoscope is passed down to the larynx; a collagen-primed needle is passed through the cricothyroid membrane, into the subglottic area, and infiltrates the vocal cords from below. The surgeon is able to see the bulking effect on the television monitor and obtain feedback of phonation from the fully conscious patient. The primary disadvantage of this procedure is that there is a limited access to the anterior glottis due to the curvature of the transcricoid needle. Furthermore the "operator" does not directly visualize the point of injection, as it is underneath the cord. The injection from an inferior point also causes the bulking effect of the vocal cord to the inferior surface rather than the more optimal superior surface.

Transnasal laryngoesophagoscopy (TNLE) facilitates vocal cord injection under direct vision and under local anesthetic, with the advantages of the previously described methods without their disadvantages. There are no restrictions on the placement of the needle; the anterior commissure is easily reached. Injection can be performed in an accurate and controlled manner to the superior surface of the cords. The technique is performed under local anesthetic, so the patient is able to give feedback and it is tolerated well by the patient (described in other chapters).

Direct phonoplasty with TNLE is effective, well tolerated, safe, and can be performed in the outpatients department or day-case surgery unit (Video 12).

METHOD
The consented patient is prepared with local anesthesia as previously described. Further local anesthetic (2% lignocaine) may be dripped directly onto the cords via an epidural catheter passed down the instrument channel.

The endoscope is passed transnasal to the larynx, where the vocal cords may be visualized on a television monitor. The 23-gauge endoscopic needle, pre-primed with collagen for injection, is passed down the instrument channel (Fig. 4.2.1). The authors use collagen; however, alternative materials such as Teflon or Gelfoam may also be used.

Under direct vision of the paralyzed vocal cords, the surgeon is then able to inject directly into the superior surface of the cords (Fig. 4.2.2).

The collagen is injected precisely, lateral to the cord until it lies in the desired position (Fig. 4.2.3). It is important to inject into the correct plane. Too deep an infiltration may not medialize the cord, but may narrow the subglottis. Too superficial one may obliterate the laryngeal ventricle and not medialize the cord. Medially placed injections can potentially disrupt the vibrating edge of the cord to the detriment of voice quality.

The patient phonates, allowing immediate feedback for the desired amount of collagen required. A second injection

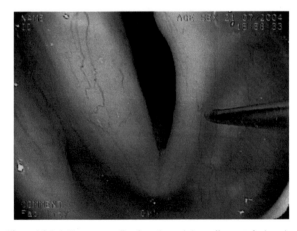

Figure 4.2.1 A 23-gauge needle advancing to inject collagen at the junction of anterior and middle thirds of paralyzed left vocal cord.

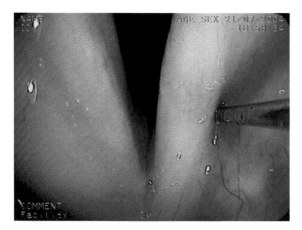

Figure 4.2.2 The injection is made lateral to the true cord.

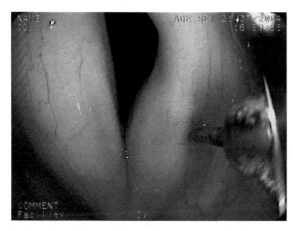

Figure 4.2.3 Collagen injected laterally bulks up the cord and moves the leading edge medially to meet the right cord.

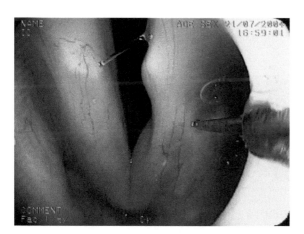

Figure 4.2.4 The needle is withdrawn and moved posteriorly to augment the posterior third of the vocal cord.

may be performed if necessary more posteriorly (Fig. 4.2.4). The posterior third of the cord can therefore be bulked up (Fig. 4.2.5).

The results of the procedure are instantaneous, with the patient's voice subjectively improving, which allows feedback as to the amount of collagen to be injected. The good apposition of the cords may also be seen on the digital monitor (Fig. 4.2.6).

Performed under local anesthetic, the patient is able to eat and drink as normal soon after the effects of the local anesthetic have worn off, and is able to be discharged soon afterward.

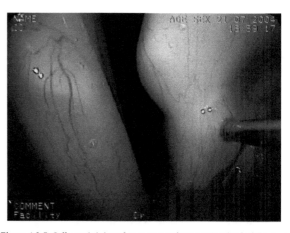

Figure 4.2.5 Collagen is injected to augment the posterior third of the cord.

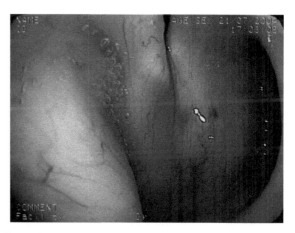

Figure 4.2.6 Complete closure of the phonatory gap after injection with very good voice production, cough, and airway protection. *Source:* (P Montgomery, A Sharma, A Qayyum and K Mierzwa. Direct phonoplasty under local anaesthetic The Journal of Laryngology & Otology, Volume 119, Issue 02, Feb 2005, pp 134–137).

4.3   TNLE and tracheoesophageal puncture
James Snelling

Vocal rehabilitation following laryngectomy has long been a challenge. Throughout the history of laryngectomy there are reports of successful voice production with either planned or serendipitous spontaneous fistulae. Unfortunately, most early attempts to surgically fashion fistulae to allow exhaled air to pass between the trachea and pharynx produced inconsistent voice and were commonly compromised by salivary leak.

The current mainstay of surgical voice restoration post laryngectomy is tracheoesophageal puncture and voice prosthesis placement. This gold standard treatment has been enormously successful since it was first described by Singer and Blom in 1980. Most tracheoesophageal punctures are performed primarily but there are still clinical situations where a secondary puncture is prudent. Secondary puncture is now mainly reserved for patients following pharyngolaryngectomy or partial pharyngectomy and complex reconstruction, primarily because of concern regarding the risk of breakdown and unintended fistula formation within the posterior tracheal wall. Secondary puncture is also indicated for the revision of a problematic primary puncture.

Surgical voice restoration using the secondary tracheoesophageal puncture has traditionally been performed under general anesthetic in an operating theatre with a rigid esophagoscope. This has the disadvantages of requirement for inpatient or day-case surgical admission as well as the risk of adverse events associated with anesthesia or the use of rigid instrumentation.

Secondary tracheoesophageal puncture and speech valve insertion can be performed under local anesthetic in the outpatient department with a transnasal laryngoesophagoscope (TNLE) with a 2.0-mm operating channel to assist the procedure (video 13).

The pharynx is prepared in the standardized fashion described earlier. The patient is positioned sitting up and the party wall anesthetized by local infiltration through the stoma with 2 ml of 1% lignocaine. The endoscope is passed transnasally and the upper esophageal segment is insufflated with air allowing excellent visualization of the anterior pharyngeal wall. Puncture is made with a cannula and the tract is subsequently dilated with a series of dilating probes followed by the appropriate voice prosthesis dilator. The tract is subsequently measured and an appropriately sized speaking valve is inserted. The procedure is outlined in Fig. 4.3.1.

The utilization of TNLE allows insufflation of the pharynx and thereby a direct observation of the procedure. Risk of damage to the posterior esophageal wall is thus minimized. The excellent pharyngeal view also allows early identification of problems during this procedure that might otherwise go unnoticed, resulting in problems. In Figure 4.3.2, one can see how a false tract can be identified promptly, preventing a subsequent potentially traumatic manipulation of the tracheoesophageal segment.

The images shown here illustrate the insertion of a nonindwelling, low pressure voice prosthesis but the technique would be equally applicable to an indwelling prosthesis.

In conclusion, the TNLE enables a simple and safe technique for the insertion of a voice prosthesis. The procedure is comfortably tolerated by the subject such that the surgical voice restoration can be performed in the outpatient department without the need for general anesthesia.

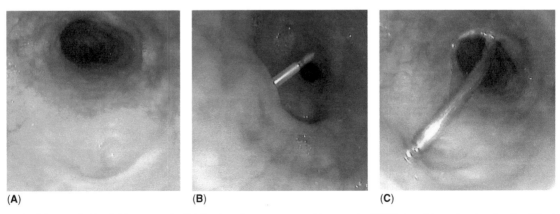

(A)   **(B)**   **(C)**

Figure 4.3.1 (A) View of a closed old puncture site. (B) Creation of a new puncture with a cannula. (C) Dilation with a series of steel probes. (*Continued*)

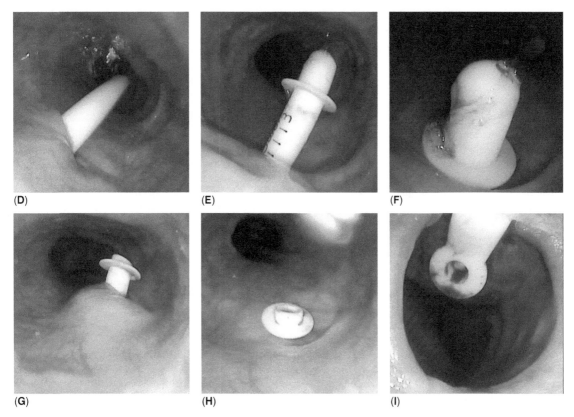

(D)   (E)   (F)

(G)   (H)   (I)

Figure 4.3.1 (*Continued*) (**D**) Dilatation with a Blom-Singer 16 Fr dilator (InHealth Technologies, Carpinteria, USA). (**E**) Insertion of a sizing device. (**F**) Sizing of the tract. (**G**) Low pressure nonindwelling prosthesis insertion. (**H**) Final internal appearance. (**I**) Final external appearance.   *Source*: Snelling JD, Price T, Montgomery PQ, Blagnys BL. How we do it: Secondary trache-oesophageal puncture under local anaesthetic, using a trans-nasal flexible laryngo-esophagoscope (TNFLO). Logopedics Phoniatrics Vocology 2006 Online.

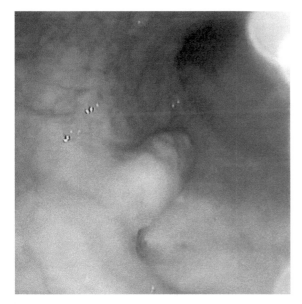

Figure 4.3.2 Identification of a false passage created while dilating the tract.   *Source*: Same as that in the other figure.

5.1　Total laryngectomy: Primary and flap repair

Animesh J. Patel and Jonothan J. Clibbon

INTRODUCTION

Owing in part to the functional morbidity of the extirpative surgery, and advances in laser treatment and chemoradiotherapy, there has been an increasing shift toward the use of larynx-preserving treatment in patients with laryngeal cancers. As a consequence, total laryngectomy is often reserved for patients who suffer tumor recurrence after chemoradiation (salvage laryngectomy). Total laryngectomy is also a first-line treatment in patients who have very advanced tumors with invasion into adjacent structures, where primary chemoradiotherapy is deemed inappropriate. Compared to primary laryngectomy, salvage laryngectomy has been associated with significantly higher rates of perioperative and postoperative complications, mainly due to poor local tissue quality, and hence poor healing, as a consequence of the radiotherapy.

A key component of total laryngectomy is the restoration of a functional swallowing mechanism. The intimate anatomical relationship of the larynx and pharynx necessitates at least a partial pharyngectomy. The position and extent of the tumor will dictate the exact surgical excision margins and, in turn, the possibility of primary pharyngeal closure. Tumor characteristics and staging, as well as previous chemoradiation, will also determine the need for pedicled or free flaps as part of the reconstruction.

LARYNGECTOMY WITH PRIMARY REPAIR

This surgery is reserved for the relatively small primary tumor, with no extralaryngeal extension. In these cases, a small portion of the anterior pharyngeal wall may need to be resected depending on the nature of the primary tumor. There must be sufficient pharyngeal mucosa after resection to allow complete direct closure over a nasogastric tube with a lumen of at least 1 cm at the distal end. At this stage it is appropriate to insert a vocal rehabilitation prosthesis to enable subsequent tracheo-esophageal speech.

The repair of the pharynx must be in at least two layers and must be completely tension-free. Adequate pharyngeal closure is vital in minimizing the risk of dehiscence and subsequent fistula formation, one of the more common early complications of this surgery.

Where possible, if direct closure is undertaken, all efforts to maximize wound healing should be made. The patient's nutritional status should be optimized, and during surgery careful tissue handling is paramount. Meticulous hemostasis is essential and a closed suction drainage method should be used postoperatively to minimize fluid collections. Any compromise can result in excessive fluid collection around the repair site, which in turn can lead to wound breakdown and fistula formation.

LARYNGECTOMY WITH FLAP REPAIR

As the risk of pharyngocutaneous fistula formation is significantly higher in patients undergoing salvage surgery following prior chemoradiation, plastic surgeons look to employ additional reconstructive techniques to supplement the pharyngeal closure. As such, it is generally considered good practice to provide a layer of healthy, well-vascularized, nonirradiated tissue over the pharyngeal repair. This can be achieved by using regional pedicled flaps or distant-free flaps and these manoeuvres increase the chances of primary wound healing at the pharyngeal repair site. A flap may also be required in the event of there being an external skin defect following tumor resection, and such reconstruction can be achieved using a flap with a skin paddle or alternatively a muscle flap with an overlying skin graft.

A flap is defined as a block of tissue that is transferred from one part of the body to another, and the tissue brings its blood supply with it (as opposed to a graft which is reliant on its recipient site for nutrition and revascularization). A pedicled flap is one in which the blood supply remains intact during movement to its recipient site. In contrast, a free flap's blood supply (its pedicle) is divided at its donor site and then reanastomosed to blood vessels at the recipient site, using microsurgery. As the blood supply of a pedicled flap is not interrupted, the chances of flap failure are minimal. However, in free-tissue transfer, re-establishing the blood supply with microvascular surgery carries the inherent risk of vessel anastomotic problems, which could lead to flap failure. Hence, free flaps have a higher risk of failure compared to pedicled flaps. However, the main advantages of using free flaps include harvesting flaps from sites where donor morbidity is minimal and allowing a two-team approach of simultaneous tumor resection and flap harvest, thus minimizing overall operative time.

Pedicled Flaps (e.g. Pectoralis Major Muscle) vs. Musculocutaneous Flaps

Traditionally, before the advent of free tissue transfer, the pectoralis major myocutaneous flap was used extensively in this setting (Fig. 5.1.1). This robust and relatively easily raised flap is ideally suited to the task described. The pectoralis major flap was described by Ariyan in 1979, and has since become a workhorse in head and neck reconstruction. In the context of laryngopharyngeal reconstruction, the flap can be used as a muscle-only flap or as a musculocutaneous flap.

The pectoralis major muscle comprises a sternocostal head and a clavicular head which both converge to attach on the proximal humerus. It has a very reliable blood supply, from the pectoral branch of the thoracoacromial trunk with additional

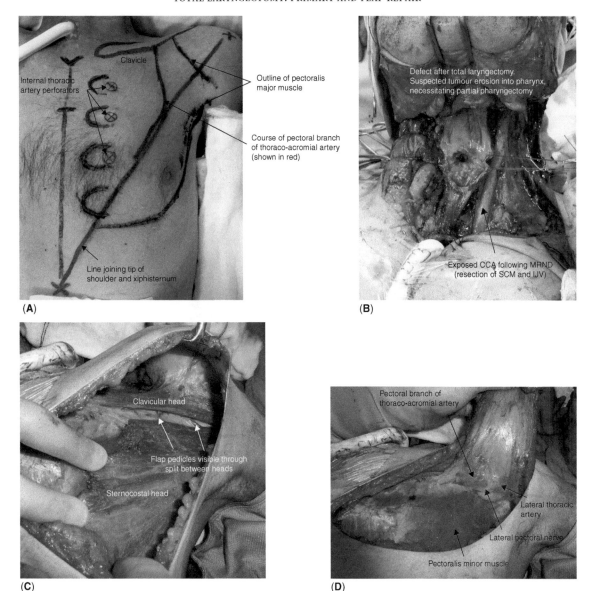

Figure 5.1.1 Pectoralis muscle flap for coverage of laryngectomy defect. The patient is a 43-year old with a radio-recurrent transglottic squamous cell car-cinoma. The patient underwent total laryngectomy, partial pharyngectomy, left neck lymphadenectomy, and coverage with a pedicled pectoralis major muscle flap. (A) Initial markings. A vertical line is drawn from the midpoint of the clavicle and continues down an oblique line drawn from the tip of the shoulder to the xiphisternum, as shown in red. This marks the flap's main pedicle. The upper internal thoracic artery perforators are marked. (B) Defect following resection. Primary closure of the pharyngeal defect was possible. *Abbreviations*: CCA, common carotid artery; IJV, internal jugular vein; MRND, modified radical neck dissection; SCM, sternocleidomastoid. (C) The 2 heads of the pectoralis major muscle. The sternocostal head must be divided lateral to the internal thoracic perforators. These vessels need to be preserved to supply a deltopectoral flap, if required. (D) The vascular pedicles of the pectoralis major muscle flap, seen on the underside of the flap. (*Continued*)

supply from the lateral thoracic artery and from perforators from the internal thoracic artery. For use in the laryngectomy patient, it is raised principally on the pectoral branch of the thoracoacromial artery (the lateral thoracic artery can also be included), which is present on the undersurface of the mus-cle, and extreme care must be taken not to damage it during flap elevation.

The skin incision used is the so-called "defensive" approach (originally described by McGregor) and this incision, com-bined with preservation of the upper internal thoracic artery perforators, provides the option of using the deltopectoral flap should it be required at a later time.

When raising the pectoralis major flap, typically only the sternocostal portion is required. Once raised, the flap is turned

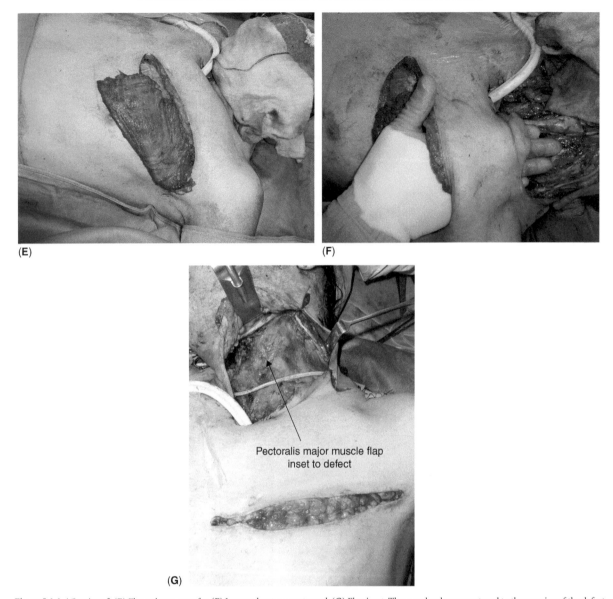

Figure 5.1.1 (*Continued*) (E) Flap prior to transfer. (F) Large subcutaneous tunnel. (G) Flap inset. The muscle edges are sutured to the margins of the defect and, in this case, the muscle covers the pharyngeal repair site and the exposed carotid artery.

over the clavicle to reach the neck and, if necessary, the clavicular head can be divided. This facilitates a greater movement of the flap, minimizes the bulge of the muscle bulk over the clavicle, and allows the muscle flap to sit comfortably. In order to transpose the muscle to the neck, a sufficiently large subcutaneous tunnel must be developed, and this must be large enough to not compress the muscle's vascular pedicle. As long as the flap is raised with care and inset tension-free without any pressure on the vascular pedicle, the risks of flap failure are minimal.

When the tumor extirpation has necessitated the resection of part of the anterior pharyngeal wall and primary closure is not possible, the flap can be raised with a skin paddle to reconstruct the pharyngeal defect. If a direct closure of the pharynx is possible, a muscle-only pectoralis flap can be used to cover the pharyngeal suture line.

When raising a musculocutaneous flap, extra care must be taken to minimize the shearing forces on the skin paddle. The actual perforating vessels that supply the overlying skin paddle are delicate and shearing can be minimized by anchoring the edge of the skin paddle to the underlying muscle.

Patients with Poland's sequence may have congenital absence of the pectoralis muscles, but otherwise the flap can be raised in both sexes and in patients of all ages. As it is a significant accessory muscle of respiration, the implications of its use in patients with pre-existing cardiac or respiratory diseases must be considered. Harvesting the pectoralis major muscle may affect breathing in these patients, increasing the risks of pulmonary morbidity and where necessary an alternative flap should be used.

Free Flaps

In the last few decades, with improvements in microsurgical expertise and better understanding of vascular anatomy, the emergence of free tissue transfer has revolutionized reconstructive surgery. In the context of the head and neck oncology patient, potential flaps that can be used include muscle flaps, fasciocutaneous flaps, and composite flaps that contain bone, muscle, and skin.

Muscle-Free Flaps (e.g., Gracilis)

For the laryngectomy patient in whom a primary pharyngeal closure is possible, a muscle-only flap will suffice to cover the pharyngeal suture line. In our unit, our first choice is the gracilis muscle. The gracilis is a thin, long muscle that forms part of the adductor compartment of the thigh. It originates at the inferior pubic ramus and inserts distally as a long tendon to the medial upper tibia. It has a dominant vascular supply, the adductor branch of the profunda femoris, located in the proximal third of the muscle (this is often confused with the medial circumflex femoral artery), supplemented by secondary minor vascular

pedicles more distally. The proximal part of the muscle is all that is necessary, and the tendinous part is generally not needed. Following harvest, donor site morbidity is minimal. The flap can be raised as a musculocutaneous flap, but the reliability of the skin paddle is variable and careful planning is required to ensure the presence of adequate perforators to it.

Fasciocutaneous Free Flaps

When pharyngeal closure is tight or when there is an external skin defect, the anterolateral thigh flap or the radial forearm free flap can provide tissue with a skin paddle. The anterolateral thigh fasciocutaneous flap is based on perforators from the descending branch of the lateral circumflex femoral artery. If a small skin paddle is raised, the donor site can be closed directly to leave an acceptable linear scar with minimal donor site morbidity. The radial forearm free flap is based on septocutaneous perforators from the radial artery. The main drawback of this flap is that the donor site usually requires a skin graft to close it, and this can leave a cosmetically poor scar. Arterial dominance to the hand must always be tested using the Allen's test, prior to raising a radial forearm flap to ensure the hand will be adequately perfused after harvest of the radial artery.

SUMMARY

The selection of the method of closure, be it direct closure or with flap cover, depends on the nature of the surgery and the resultant defect and must be decided on an individual-patient basis. In the salvage laryngectomy patient, the main objective is to bring healthy, well-vascularized tissue into an area that has been previously treated with radiotherapy to maximize the chances of primary wound healing and minimize the risk of pharyngocutaneous fistula.

5.2 Flap monitoring

Animesh J. Patel and Jonothan J. Clibbon

INTRODUCTION

The rationale behind flap monitoring is to be able to provide timely and appropriate interventions to flaps that are of questionable viability or impending necrosis. In the first 24–48 hours after surgery, flaps should be closely monitored by experienced staff and flap observations need to be recorded at least hourly. Any change in the flap's clinical status should activate a system incorporating senior review and immediate return to the operating theater where necessary. Hence, reconstructive surgery with the use of flaps should only be undertaken in units where these systems are in place and there is sufficient clinical expertise to recognize and effectively manage compromised flaps.

Patients undergoing complicated reconstructive surgery after laryngectomy often need to be nursed in a high-dependency facility in the early postoperative period. During this time, as well as regular flap monitoring, the patient must be assessed as a whole, with accurate regular recording of respiratory and haemodynamic parameters. Oxygen saturations, respiratory rate, pulse rate, systemic blood pressure, temperature, and hourly urine output measurements must be recorded, and any deviation from normal should be addressed. Urine output is an accurate, noninvasive measure of fluid balance in patients undergoing reconstructive surgery, and in the case of free-flap surgery, aiming for a urine output of 1 ml/kg/hr is necessary to maintain the hyperdynamic circulation that the flap requires.

MONITORING OF PEDICLED FLAPS

Most of the pedicled flaps used routinely in head and neck surgery are robust, with a good blood supply, and infrequently suffer from vascular problems. Very occasionally a poorly perfused portion of a flap, typically the distal tip that is furthest from the flap's blood supply (pedicle), may undergo necrosis. Problems in pedicled flaps usually stem from excessive external pressure on the pedicle and so long as this is recognized in a timely fashion, pedicled flaps will usually survive such insults.

MONITORING OF FREE FLAPS

Free tissue transfer is a complex and technically demanding enterprise that inherently carries the risk of vascular compromise. Problems relating to the arterial and venous microanastomoses can translate into complete ischemia and subsequent necrosis of the entire flap. Flap death is usually an all-or-nothing event and if it does occur, represents significant additional morbidity for the patient.

Monitoring of Cutaneous/Myocutaneous Flaps

Flaps that have been fashioned to include a skin paddle are readily monitored by assessing certain key clinical parameters, which can be achieved through inspection, palpation, and auscultation. Assessment of a flap's skin paddle is one of the most accurate and reliable methods of ascertaining adequate perfusion of the flap as a whole, but must be done by appropriately trained staff.

Key features visible to the naked eye include the colour and capillary return time, and palpation of the flap's skin paddle that will allow assessment of skin temperature and turgor, as well as the presence of swelling or hematoma, either of which could potentially compromise the flap. This is true for either pedicled flaps or free flaps; yet, it should be noted that pedicled flaps can become slightly more congested than free flaps without any detriment.

A healthy skin paddle will be of normal skin color (relative to the part of the body it has been transferred from), will have a capillary return time of ~2 seconds, will be warm to touch and be soft in its consistency.

The presence of perforating blood vessels in the flap's skin paddle will allow the auscultation of arterial and venous signals with a hand-held Doppler probe, and in such cases it is useful to mark the site of skin perforators with a suture to facilitate postoperative monitoring. Hand-held Doppler probes are particularly useful for monitoring the skin paddle in flaps that are especially pale, such as the anterolateral thigh flap. Ultrasound energy is emitted by the Doppler probe and reflected from moving red blood cells, which is then picked up by the probe and heard as an audible signal. A satisfactory venous signal will be heard as a monophasic waveform, and a pulsatile biphasic signal will be heard with a patent artery. One significant downside of relying on auscultation of an arterial signal is that there can be a delay of up to 5 hours between an onset of venous obstruction and a loss of the arterial Doppler signal. Hence, a combined clinical assessment and Doppler auscultation is essential.

Monitoring of Buried Flaps and Adjuncts to Monitoring

Any flap that has no visible portion because of its design is more difficult to monitor. A pectoralis major flap with a skin paddle resurfacing the pharynx may have no skin paddle on direct view. Similarly, reconstructions using free tissue such as jejunum or a tubed anterolateral thigh flap cannot be monitored by traditional means. In such circumstances, monitor segments can be raised from the 'parent' flap and brought to a visible location in order to more easily assess viability of the whole construct.

New technological advances have also provided additional monitoring aids. Implantable Doppler probes can be used to monitor the arterial supply and/or the venous output. The Cook–Swartz implantable Doppler device, as shown in Figure 5.2.1, can

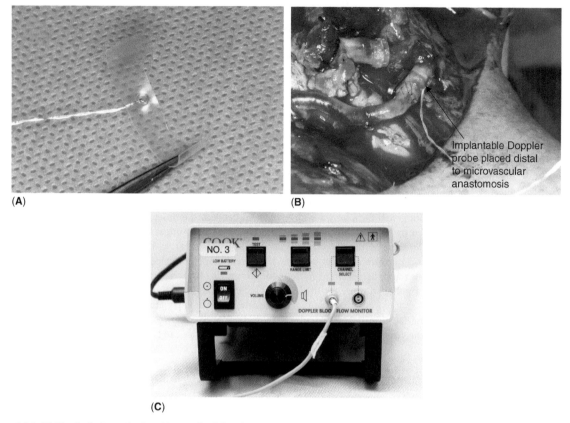

Figure 5.2.1 (**A**) The Cook–Swartz implantable Doppler. (**B**) A close-up view of Doppler flow probe cuff *in situ*, placed on a vessel distal to the microvascular anastomosis (**C**) Doppler blood flow monitor. Cook–Swartz Doppler Flow Monitoring System courtesy of Cook Medical, Cook Ireland Ltd, Limerick, Ireland.

be placed on either the artery or vein. Early experience with the placement of the device on the artery revealed a 3–5% false-positive rate in terms of loss of signal that resulted in unnecessary flap re-explorations and a similar false-negative rate, resulting in flap failure. Placement of the probe on the vein has been shown to be more accurate, with minimal delay in loss of signal from time of onset of vessel obstruction. Although implantable Doppler probes can prove invaluable in monitoring buried flaps, they are not available in all units and are also associated with a significant cost.

Other adjuncts to monitoring flaps include the use of laser Doppler, oxygen partial pressure probes, thermal diffusion probes, and biochemical microdialysis probes. These technologies are not readily available, but have shown encouraging results where they have been used.

IDENTIFYING A FAILING FLAP

The reasons for which free flaps fail are numerous. Whatever the cause, the final common endpoint is thrombosis at the site of the microsurgical anastomosis.

Pre-/Intraoperative Error

Successful flap surgery starts long before the operation. It is important that a flap is planned well; the correct flap must be selected to do a particular task and it must be inset to the surgical defect in a way that causes no embarrassment of its own circulation. Flaps that are raised inexpertly, with insufficient knowledge of the surgical anatomy or with careless dissection around the vascular pedicle may be doomed from the outset. Once raised, meticulous technique is essential for a successful microvascular anastomosis. A suboptimal anastomosis can result in damage to the blood vessel intima and cause abnormal flow disturbances that will increase the chances of platelet aggregation and thrombosis formation.

Arterial Insufficiency

Flaps must have an adequate arterial inflow in order to perfuse the tissues raised. Inadequate inflow will lead to ischemia, followed by necrosis, if not recognized and treated. Arterial problems in flaps commonly arise due to thrombosis of the arterial microanastomosis, or kinking or external compression of the pedicle. Flaps with arterial insufficiency generally have a pale appearance, are flaccid and either do not bleed or bleed very slowly when pricked with a needle.

Problems with inflow can also be a result of hemodynamic instability. The patient who is underfilled as a whole, reflected in hypotension and poor urine output, may also be unable to adequately perfuse the flap, and hence adequate fluid management in the early postoperative period is essential.

Venous Insufficiency

Just as important as inflow, the flap must have an adequate venous outflow to avoid congestion, swelling, and ultimately, death. Flap congestion is caused by thrombus of the venous microanastomosis, clot propagation or twisting, and kinking or pressure on the vascular pedicle. Congested flaps have a swollen, tense feel and take on a mottled or purplish-blue appearance. When pricked with a needle, there is usually a rapid appearance of dark blood. Extrinsic pressure can also result from hematomas and tight dressings and, as veins are more compressible than arteries, can be a potential cause for inadequate venous outflow.

A small hematoma in the wrong location near a vascular pedicle may be enough to restrict the venous outflow of a flap.

Venous congestion may lead to secondary haemorrhage of a raised flap, and a further hematoma may ensue.

Tight dressings, clothing, and particularly retention tapes for endotracheal tubes may cause sufficient pressure to reduce or even halt blood flow in the pedicle of a flap. The same problem can also occur in pedicled flaps where the pedicle passes through a tunnel that is too tight. All such external causes of pressure should be recognized and corrected and the flap should be observed for changes.

SUMMARY

A prompt surgical exploration of a failing flap is essential to maximize the chances of flap survival. The success of such interventions in terms of flap salvage is inversely proportional to the time elapsed between the onset of flap ischemia and re-exploration. Hence, close monitoring is essential in the postoperative period.

Clinical assessment, with simple adjuncts such as the use of a hand-held Doppler device, remains the most reliable method for monitoring flaps that are visible externally. Often, flaps used for reconstruction of laryngectomy defects are buried, making the assessment of flap viability difficult. In these circumstances, in the case of free flap reconstructions, the use of an implantable Doppler device can be very useful.

5.3 Flap necrosis and postoperative fistula
Jonothan J. Clibbon and Animesh J. Patel

INTRODUCTION

The viability of a reconstructive flap is reliant on adequate blood flow into and out of the flap tissue and hence flap failure can be broadly classified into problems with arterial inflow or venous outflow. The flow in a flap's pedicle can be compromised if there is a decrease in the volume of the blood flow, thrombosis in the vessel, or if there is external compression of the artery or vein.

MANAGING THE FAILING FLAP

In the first instance, the patient must be assessed as a whole. Inadequate perfusion may be a result of overall hypotension, which should be aggressively managed with intravenous fluids to ensure an adequate blood flow into the flap. Prompt release of any tight dressings or sutures may help alleviate compression on the flap's pedicle. Similarly, if a hematoma is suspected, a prompt evacuation is necessary to prevent further compromise to the flap. Other causes of pedicle compression include kinking due to poor alignment of the pedicle intraoperatively or stretching of a pedicle. In free flaps, if there is any suspicion of flap compromise, then the possibility of thrombosis at the site of the microvascular anastomoses should be considered and urgent re-exploration of the flap's pedicle, with resuturing of the microvascular anastomoses, will be necessary.

Flap Necrosis in Pedicled Flaps

Occasionally, the pedicled myocutaneous flap will undergo necrosis of the skin paddle, as shown in Figure 5.3.1. This is usually because there has been insufficient care during flap elevation, or the skin paddle has insufficient perforating vessels to allow an adequate perfusion. It is uncommon for the pedicled flap to undergo total necrosis, unless the pedicle is damaged during flap elevation or if the flap is inset with too much tension or kinking of the pedicle.

Flap Necrosis in Free Flaps

Despite good monitoring practices and appropriate timely interventions, up to 5% of free flaps may fail completely. In free tissue transfers, the loss is in the vast majority of cases total, as by definition, there is no collateral supply. Occasionally, very large free flaps lose a small distal portion.

Free flap failure shows a biphasic distribution. Early failure tends to be due to technical problems at the site of the microvascular anastomoses, and can present any time in the first week. Late failures, after one week, are much less common and are most often due to infective causes.

SIGNS OF FLAP NECROSIS

Depending on the purpose of the flap, the loss of the flap can potentially be disastrous for the surgical outcome. During the first 24–48 hours, following the cessation of circulation in a flap, it is not always entirely obvious on inspection that a problem exists. Hence, monitoring by trained staff is essential to pick up potential problems early.

In two to five days, the tissues of the flap start to undergo liquefactive necrosis, accompanied by a characteristic foul smell, skin changes, and wound dehiscence, which in turn leads to fistula formation.

TREATMENT OF FLAP NECROSIS

The result of flap necrosis is obviously highly dependent on the anatomical location and extent of the necrosis. In laryngeal surgery and pharyngeal reconstruction, flap failure will tend to result in the formation of a pharyngocutaneous fistula. A large area of flap loss will clearly increase the chance of a large fistula whereas a minor flap edge dehiscence will likely result in a small fistula. As a general principle, necrotic tissue should be debrided and replaced with further fresh flap tissue.

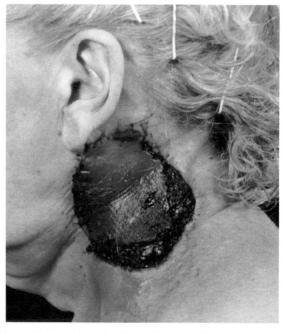

Figure 5.3.1 Necrosis of the skin paddle of a pedicled pectoralis major myocutaneous flap.

PHARYNGOCUTANEOUS FISTULAE

One of the major challenges of laryngectomy/pharyngectomy and subsequent reconstruction is fistula prevention and management. The reasons for fistula development are often multifactorial. Preoperative considerations include any general factors that may compromise wound healing and include nutritional status, anemia, diabetes, and cigarette smoking. One of the main contributing factors is preoperative chemoradiotherapy.

The rate of fistula formation in primary laryngeal repair with no previous radiotherapy is approximately 10%, although rates do vary between centers. This rate rises dramatically in the presence of previous chemoradiotherapy to 30% and in some centers, up to 50% rates are reported.

Early Fistula Formation

Early fistula formation is normally the result of suboptimal perioperative management. In order to minimize the incidence of early fistulae, meticulous surgical technique with atraumatic handling of tissues is essential. Closure of the pharyngeal defect must be tension-free to achieve a watertight suture line, ideally as two layers. These patients often undergo a simultaneous cervical lymphadenectomy; therefore, meticulous hemostasis is necessary to prevent hematoma formation, as is the use of closed-suction drainage in the immediate postoperative period to minimize seroma.

Despite the best efforts, fistulae do occur and in such circumstances, patients should be managed by a strict nil-by-mouth regime for up to two weeks. During this time, nutrition should be replaced by nasogastric or gastrostomy feeding. At the end of the initial period, patency of the neopharynx (surgically reconstructed pharynx) and the presence of fistulae can be observed by barium swallow investigation, as shown in Figure 5.3.2. Fistulae that do arise in this period commonly drain onto the skin or create a blind-ending pouch or pocket.

Early fistulae are often small and a majority of these can be managed nonsurgically and will close spontaneously with conservative measures. During this time, these patients require meticulous wound care, appropriate wound dressings, and topical or systemic antibiotics. Also, they will require a further period of restricted oral intake, with adequate nutritional support.

Larger fistulae can also be managed conservatively in the first instance. However, if there is little evidence of healing, or if the fistula is associated with a significant soft tissue defect, then consideration should be given to further surgical intervention. This will involve debridement of any nonviable tissue and interposing either a regional pedicled flap or a distant free flap. If such a flap was used in the primary procedure, the viability of the flap must be assessed and if debridement is necessary, another flap will need to be used.

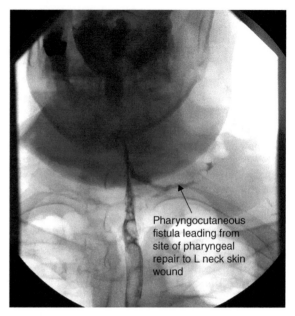

Figure 5.3.2 Barium swallow investigation illustrating the presence of a pharyngocutaneous fistula.

Late Fistula Formation

Most of the early postsurgical fistulae do not require intervention and close spontaneously. However, delayed formation may represent a problem with the healing of the neopharynx. This may be due to the effects of radiotherapy on the tissues or flap problems. In some cases, it is a sign of recurrent disease, and this must always be excluded in fistulae that show minimal signs of healing. Late fistulae tend not to fully close spontaneously and can also open to surfaces other than skin. Surgical intervention, with further reconstructive procedures, is often required to manage these problems and accurate diagnosis with barium investigation is useful.

SUMMARY

Previous chemoradiotherapy is an independent risk factor for the development of pharyngocutaneous fistula following total laryngectomy. Tissues that have been exposed to radiation are often of poor quality, and combined with systemic factors such as poor nutrition, patients' wound healing capabilities are compromised. If the pedicled or free flaps that have been used in the primary surgery fail, fistula formation is inevitable. When they do occur, the majority can be managed nonsurgically, but require meticulous wound care as well as sufficient nutritional support. Large fistulae, or fistulae that do not heal with conservative measures, need debridement of nonviable tissue and further reconstructive surgery.

5.4 Surgical voice restoration
Gill Faley, Karyn Stewart-Dodd, and Sue Trim

INTRODUCTION

The most commonly used form of speech restoration post laryngectomy is surgical voice restoration (SVR).

It is regarded as the optimum method for voice restoration aiming to have as-near normal speech as is possible, within two to three weeks of surgery.

Laryngectomy surgery involves the separation of the respiratory and vocal tracts. The actual voice-producing mechanism, the larynx incorporating the vocal folds, is removed.

There is no longer any way that the airflow from the lungs can reach the mouth to be modified by the articulators to form speech sounds. Nor is there any mechanism now to produce voice in order to make speech audible.

SVR creates a tract or fistula between the trachea and the esophagus, maintained by the use of a voice prosthesis, to enable air to be directed from the lungs through the tract and into the esophagus (Fig. 5.4.1).

As air directed through the tracheoesophageal tract passes up through the esophagus toward the pharynx, it generates vibrations in the pharyngoesophageal (PE) segment. The vibrations give the supporting sound to make speech audible, that is, voice.

The air pressure necessary to make this voice is achieved by the patients occluding the stoma through which they breathe, at the time that they wish to divert air from the lungs and trachea, through a one-way valve into the esophagus and onward and upward for voice and speech.

The air travels from the lungs, into the esophagus and up through the PE segment and vocal tract. The sound produced resonates in the vocal tract and the speech articulators modify the airflow to create speech sounds.

It is necessary, however, to ensure that when the patient eats and drinks, food and liquid do not flow back through the newly created tract between esophagus and trachea, and down into the lungs.

To prevent this happening, the voice prosthesis has a one-way valve. The valve allows air from the lungs to be diverted through the tract as a result of occlusion of the stoma but prevents food and liquid flowing back through it (Fig. 5.4.2).

THE BENEFITS OF SVR

SVR is, as has already been said, the optimum method for voice restoration post laryngectomy, for most patients.

The benefits of SVR over other methods of speech production as listed below:

- Voicing is louder.
- Longer sentences can be achieved on one breath.
- Patients generally acquire speech which is easily intelligible to the average listener, more quickly.
- Speech is more normal to the listener, incorporating improved pitch variability.
- There is no extraneous device to be remembered, used, or carried around.
- The speech produced and mode of speech tend to be psychologically more acceptable to the patient.
- The speech produced and mode of speech are generally more easily socially integrated into the general public domain.

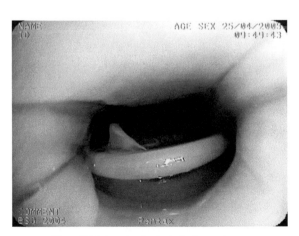

Figure 5.4.1 Speech valve *in situ* in the esophagus.

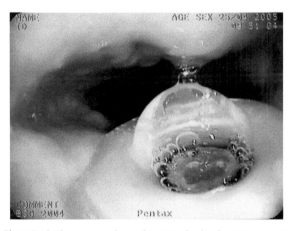

Figure 5.4.2 The one-way valve can be seen in the closed position, preventing esophageal contents leaking into the trachea.

LONG-TERM CLINICAL MANAGEMENT

SVR offers the best voicing prospects for patients in most instances but it is not always straightforward.

The aim is generally to have patients/carers independently caring for their own valves, including changing them. They can then manage cleaning the valves and leakage problems when the valve is failing, as and when they occur, without the need to visit clinics.

However, valve management can be more problematic for some patients, with a high dependency on visits to a specialist clinical service in the early stages.

Frequent problems with leakage can be caused by candida colonization of the voice prosthesis. Some patients are particularly susceptible to this. Treatment options include antifungal regimes, for example, amphotericin or nystatin or, in highly resistant cases, the use of a specialist candida-resistant valve (Figs. 5.4.3–5.4.5).

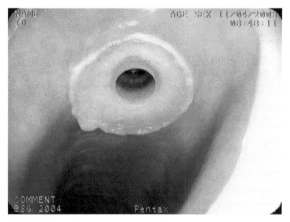

Figure 5.4.3 Candidal colonization of the rim of the valve in the trachea.

The growth of granulation tissue in or around the tract can be an issue with the potential to cover the valve opening or to alter the tract shape or size, leading to malfunction or potential displacement. Small amounts of granulation tissue can be treated with silver nitrate. Larger amounts may require laser surgery.

Stoma size needs to be monitored. If the stoma is too small, valve management is more difficult.

Sometimes the tract lumen becomes too large. There is then potential for leakage around the valve and a risk of the valve being dislodged. Alternatively, the lumen can be small and tight, making valve changes more difficult and encompassing a risk of trauma to the tract.

The valves should be carefully fitted by experienced clinicians, as in the early stages these may need resizing at intervals as the tract size settles. They are rarely dislodged, but if this happens, a catheter or stent is required to be inserted immediately to maintain the patency of the tract and to prevent aspiration. Until such time, a fully competent clinician can fit a new valve. It is important to check that the displaced valve is not in the airway. If it is, then it must be removed. If the valve has been displaced inward into the esophagus, it will gradually move through the digestive tract. A valve that is too large can lead to pistoning in the tract and cause the growth of granulation tissue. A valve that is too small will not function properly for voicing or for prevention of aspiration and may be dislodged easily during cleaning because it is not properly secure at the back. Selecting a correct valve sizing is important.

A specialist clinical team that supports the valve users will include the consultant, a speech and language therapist, and a specialist nurse at a minimum. However, access to a dietetic, OT, physiotherapy, and psychology support is also important when considering the individual needs of the patients.

The specialist team will gradually work through any complicating issues with the patient. The patient (and carers as appropriate) will learn at a pace that suits their individual

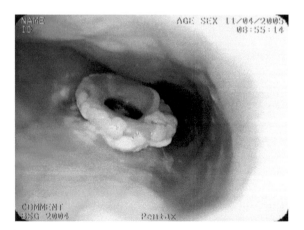

Figure 5.4.4 Internal view of the valve pictured in Fig. 5.4.3. showing mild candidal colonization.

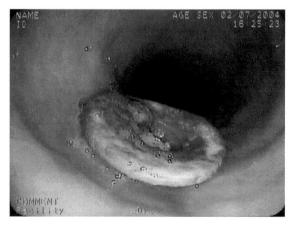

Figure 5.4.5 Heavy Candidal colonization causing a valve to leak into the trachea.

needs, how to manage the valve, and to gain confidence in their own ability to do so. They will also be taught how to voice efficiently and well.

Heat and moisture exchange systems and hands-free voicing will also be explored and implemented as appropriate under the guidance of the clinical team.

Some patients cannot self-change and do not have a carer who can change the valve for them. These patients are dependent on clinic visits for valve changes and may need to travel considerable distances to a specialist clinic. Such patients may be candidates for indwelling valves, designed to be in place longer than standard valves and to be changed by clinicians.

The multidisciplinary specialist team works closely together and with the patient, to ensure that the patient is fully informed about SVR and other communication options prior to surgery. A specialist service is essential for any patient undergoing SVR and should incorporate 24-hour access to support and advise in case of an urgent problem such as valve displacement.

ADDITIONAL CONSIDERATIONS
The following should be taken into consideration when thinking about SVR for individual patients.

- The patient's (and carer's as appropriate) views and wishes
- Manual dexterity
- Visual acuity
- Respiratory status
- PE segment function
- If alcohol or drug abuse is an issue, then a careful evaluation should be undertaken for safety reasons
- Current mode of communication if SVR is being considered some time after the original surgery. The pros and cons of change should be carefully evaluated with the patient and if appropriate, the carer.

5.5 Radiation and chemoradiation in head and neck cancer
Craig Martin

INTRODUCTION

Chemotherapy and radiotherapy are the principal nonsurgical treatment modalities used in the management of all cancers, especially in head and neck cancers. Radiotherapy alone may be the definitive management for certain tumors, for example T1 or T2 squamous carcinomas of the larynx, and radiotherapy combined with chemotherapy (chemoradiation) (CRT) is appropriate management for more advanced tumors such as squamous oropharyngeal carcinomas.

Radiotherapy may be radical (i.e., with curative intent) or palliative and may be given by external beam via a linear accelerator or by an implanted radioactive isotope such as iridium. Chemotherapy may be given prior to other cancer treatment (induction chemotherapy) methods, or in the same time-course as other treatment as in concomitant CRT, or uncommonly in HNC, following the principal treatment modality (adjuvant chemotherapy). In this chapter we discuss head and neck squamous carcinomas (HNSCC), since they account for well over 90% of head and neck cancers.

RADIOTHERAPY

Radiotherapy in HNSCC is usually radical and consists normally of daily sessions (fractions) given five times weekly to a total of 20–35 fractions. Late effects such as fibrosis or mandibular necrosis are more common with courses consisting of a smaller number of large fractions (hypofractionated radiotherapy), therefore, longer courses with 30–35 fractions each consisting of 1.8–2 Gray (Gy) over 6–7 weeks was the norm, previously. However now, it is felt that completing the radiation course within 4 weeks is more important, which results in a reduced opportunity for tumor repopulation. It is therefore now more common to use 20 fractions of 2.75 Gy each to give 55 Gy in total and complete the course in 4 weeks.

Radiotherapy produces side effects and HNSCC patients need much encouragement in order to complete their radiation course satisfactorily. These may be systemic, with fatigue, but also local, for example mucositis, as in the buccal or oropharyngeal mucosa, skin reactions, soreness on swallowing (odynophagia) leading to nutritional problems and weight loss, or salivary effects leading to dry mouth, and are discussed more fully below. Apart from causing discomfort, these reactions if not fully controlled can cause interruptions to the course of radiation treatment. Any prolongation of the overall time will run a risk of reducing the chance of curing the tumor and so is to be actively avoided.

Radiotherapy for HNSCC is precise and needs to be accurate at least to within 3 mm. In order to achieve this, a patient-specific mask ("shell") is made for the majority of these patients. This is made from Perspex (Amari Plastics, Norwich, UK) and

requires two sessions prior to the planning of the radiotherapy. Because irradiation involving the pharynx may cause dysphagia with resulting weight loss, it is important to maintain the patient's weight by means of a feeding tube inserted by gastrostomy and this is commonly inserted before the course is started. The mask has other advantages, because the planning marks can be put on the shell rather than the patient's skin, which is thus more reproducible and also better cosmetically. Radiotherapy is preferably done with 3-dimensional planning (conformal).

CHEMOTHERAPY

Chemotherapy in HNSCC usually involves a platinum agent, either cisplatin or carboplatin. Induction chemotherapy is usually given with three cycles of cisplatin and 5-fluorouracil (5FU) (PF) with response rates of over 90% and is used where there is a large tumor volume or nodal involvement so that when subsequent radiotherapy is given, the volume of tumor is smaller and the chance of cure higher. Docetaxel may be combined with PF and has been shown to increase survival, or PF alone. In addition, low-dose carboplatin can be given concomitantly with the radiotherapy with the aim of radiosensitization. In T3 or T4 tumors, where the field volume may not necessarily be large but the tumor is invading the cartilage, or in the postoperative setting, induction chemotherapy is not given but cisplatin is given concomitantly with radiotherapy.

Chemotherapy is cytotoxic and most cytotoxic agents are associated with fatigue, nausea and vomiting, and alopecia. Cisplatin alone can cause fatigue, nausea and vomiting, and renal and ototoxicity. Thus the PF regime can cause marked fatigue and emesis, although modern 5-HT3 antagonists are effective antiemetic agents. Alopecia is usually not severe with PF. At least 30% of patients will have reduced renal function after PF. Side effects from 5FU infusion include mucosal toxicity with mouth ulceration which is common and some patients with deficiency of the enzyme DPD can have severe mucositis of the small intestine, or pseudo-obstruction, which requires careful medical management in hospital. A small percentage of patients can suffer cardiac problems with angina from coronary vasospasm, myocardial infarction, hypo- or hypertension. Carboplatin, commonly used in concomitant CRT, is less emetic, nephrotoxic and ototoxic than cisplatin, but more marrow-toxic.

RADIOTHERAPY TECHNIQUES AND INDICATIONS

T1 or T2 oropharyngeal or laryngeal tumors may be treated with radiotherapy alone. T3 or T4 or node-positive oropharyngeal tumors are treated with induction and concomitant CRT and may have neck dissection subsequently unless PET scanning can show the neck to be clear. T3 laryngeal tumors are treated with CRT or surgery according to the degree of local invasion and T4 or node-positive tumors usually surgically with postoperative RT (PORT) or CRT (POCRT). Early oral cavity tumors are treated surgically, as are early paranasal sinus tumors, but later tumors are treated by surgery and PORT. Similarly, early salivary gland tumors are treated surgically and more advanced tumors with surgery and PORT. Higher-grade histology will tend to be an indication for PORT (Fig. 5.5.1A & B).

Most of the tongue tumors are treated as oral cavity tumors as discussed earlier, but tongue tumors up to around 4 cm may be treated purely by RT, using a combination of external beam RT and an implant of radioactive isotope such as iridium which may be left *in situ* for up to a few days and then removed. This has the advantage of avoiding surgery. However, this management is centralized to a few centers only, which are located often far from the patient's home. Modern surgical techniques combining partial or hemiglossectomy with a flap can leave the patient with a functioning tongue even after the resection of a large tumor, as well as good results and cosmesis. Tongue tumors of 4-mm thickness or greater if treated surgically, normally have a neck dissection, but if this is not performed, should have PORT delivered to the neck, hopefully to eradicate microscopic disease.

Indications for PORT in HNSCC may be summarized as follows:

All T3 and T4 tumors should have PORT to the primary site. Following neck dissection, where four or more nodes are involved with tumor, or where there is extracapsular spread, the neck should receive PORT. Any tumor excision with close margins, where further excision is not possible, should have PORT. There is evidence that POCRT is superior to PORT in laryngeal tumors and this is extended to apply to postoperative HNSCC settings. Higher-grade histology, (as in the paragraph "T1 or T2 oropharyngeal...") will reduce the threshold for offering PORT or POCRT.

Two special radiotherapy techniques of note in HNSCC are intensity-modulated radiotherapy (IMRT) and continuous hyperfractionated radiotherapy (CHART). IMRT is a technique which can treat awkward volumes and is used principally in two situations. (1) Radiotherapy, even conformal radiotherapy, for oropharyngeal cancer has hitherto involved irradiating the whole pharynx and nodal areas bilaterally and results in permanent mouth dryness (xerostomia). However, IMRT can treat the affected side and node areas to a high dose, while treating the contralateral side to a slightly lower dose, and effectively reduce the mean radiation dose to the contralateral parotid sufficiently, so that the xerostomia following IMRT is temporary rather than permanent (see the IMRT plan in Figure 5.5.2A & B).

(2) CHART purely involves the timing of radiotherapy, and a trial reported in 1996 which involved treating patients thrice daily for 12 consecutive days showed that similar results to conventional radiation could be achieved with reduced late toxicity.

RADIATION REACTIONS

Overall, radiotherapy is associated with acute and chronic toxicity. Radiotherapy to HNSCC can be classified according to the anatomical structure being irradiated. These commonly include the skin, mucous membrane, pharynx, larynx, salivary glands, eyes, ears, spinal cord and base of the brain. Common acute skin reactions range from faint erythema to bright erythema, leading to moist desquamation. The Radiation Therapy Oncology Group (RTOG) devised a scheme for acute radiation morbidity scoring which is especially applicable for HNSCC radiotherapy. All scores are from 0 to 4, where grade 4 is rare in most situations. For skin reactions faint erythema, bright erythema, moist desquamation in the skin are graded 1, 2, and 3 respectively while ulceration, hemorrhage, and necrosis are graded 4. Early skin reactions are helped by moisturizing creams such as aqueous cream (Figs. 5.5.3 & 5.5.4).

For most HNSCC radiotherapy, the crucial reactions which determine whether the patient will be able to cope with the treatment without it being prolonged (and therefore less biologically effective) are those in the mucous membranes, the pharynx and salivary glands, since it is these which most interfere with nutrition. For mucous membranes, the grading system

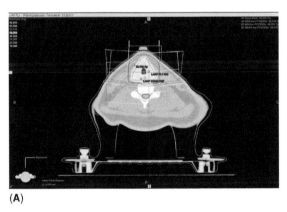

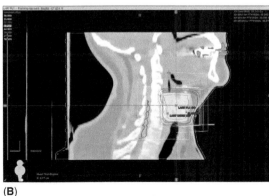

(A)   **(B)**

Figure 5.5.1 Radiotherapy plan (axial (**A**) and sagittal (**B**) views) for an early (T1b N0 M0) squamous carcinoma of right vocal cord including anterior commissure.

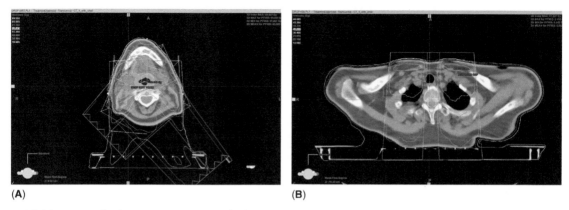

(A)   **(B)**

Figure 5.5.2 (**A**) An IMRT plan for a squamous carcinoma of right oropharynx Tx N1 M0. Five concentric beams are used to create a high-dose region including primary tumor and first-station nodal volumes on the right side, with an intermediate-dose volume to other potentially involved nodes, including contralateral nodes on the left side. (**B**) IMRT plan, same as that in (**A**). The low neck is also treated to prophylactic dose by anterior fields as above.

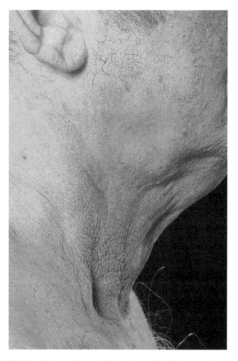

Figure 5.5.3 Grade 1 erythema of anterior neck skin in a patient receiving radiotherapy for squamous carcinoma of vocal cord T2 N0 M0.

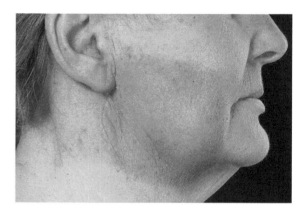

Figure 5.5.4 Grade 2 skin erythema in a patient receiving postoperative radiotherapy for carcinoma of parotid.

long-acting morphine as well, and frequently a local anesthetic spray such as Xylocaine. Hemorrhage or necrosis is again grade 4 (Figs. 5.5.5 & 5.5.6).

For the salivary glands, mild mouth dryness, thickened saliva, or a metallic taste not interfering with normal nutrition is given grade 1 and moderate to complete mouth dryness or markedly altered taste is graded 2. There is no grade 3 but grade 4 is salivary gland necrosis which is exceedingly rare. Treatment is difficult, but patients should be strongly reassured that in many situations unless salivary glands are being irradiated bilaterally, the xerostomia is temporary. Artificial saliva is disappointing, carmellose sodium (Glandosane, Freenius Kabi Ltd, Runcorn, UK.) spray has a very short-lived effect, and pilocarpine is effective only where some salivary function remains and is associated with side effects. Saliva replacement gel (Biotene OralBalance, GlaxoSmithKline, Brentford, UK.) is a new product with encouraging results. With IMRT (see the section "Radiotherapy Techniques and Indications"), the xerostomia

is based on pain and analgesic requirements: injection or mild pain not requiring analgesic is grade 1, patchy mucositis associated with moderate pain requiring analgesia is grade 2, fibrinous mucositis causing severe pain requiring a narcotic is grade 3 and ulceration. These are treated with a mouthwash such as benzydamine (Difflam), an analgesic such as paracetamol with codeine phosphate, progressing to morphine solution with

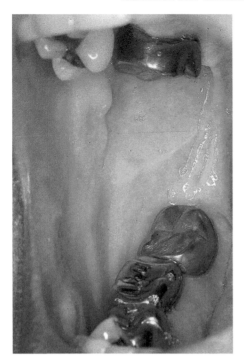

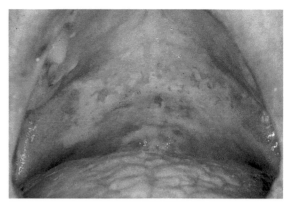

Figure 5.5.6 Fibrinous mucositis (grade 3) of the posterior pharyngeal wall and tongue in a patient receiving IMRT for squamous carcinoma of oropharynx.

Figure 5.5.5 Grade 1 mucositis of right buccal mucosa in the same patient (in Fig. 5.5.4).

following pharyngeal irradiation is reduced and, if a complete xerostomia develops in the acute phase, the patient can be reassured that it is likely to settle eventually, though this can take up to a year or two.

For the pharynx, mild dysphagia or odynophagia not requiring analgesia or topical anesthesia but allowing a soft diet is grade 1, more severe dysphagia or odynophagia requiring a narcotic or a liquid diet is grade 2, more severe reaction requiring tube feeding is grade 3 while the rare grade 4 is any case of obstruction, ulceration, perforation, or fistula. Lidocaine mixtures, often combined with steroid, can be valuable in helping patients with grade 1 or 2 pharyngitis. Grade 2 or 3 will require a narcotic and, if patients have difficulty in taking tablets or mixtures, subcutaneous fentanyl patches can produce effective pain relief. Many patients whose treatment requires that the oropharynx is irradiated bilaterally now receive gastrostomy tubes inserted proactively rather than waiting for weight loss to develop. Apart from the obvious discomfort to the patient, this can lead to the shell becoming loose, endangering the accuracy of radiotherapy.

Laryngeal reactions range from cough (grade 1) or hoarseness and sore throat but are able to vocalize (grade 2), to whispered speech, pain in throat, or referred pain to ear requiring a narcotic (grade 3) while dyspnea with stridor or hemoptysis requiring tracheostomy or intubation is grade 4. In fact, a degree of stridor from tracheal edema is not rare in HNSCC irradiation and can be controlled by dexamethasone in doses of 8–16 mg daily, but these patients require careful

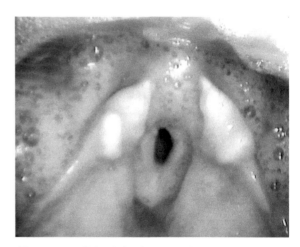

Figure 5.5.7 Radiation-induced mucositis of the larynx and pharynx.

monitoring with ENT referral if the stridor suddenly deteriorates (Fig. 5.5.7).

Acute reactions in the eye range from mild or moderate conjunctivitis (grade 1 or 2) which can be treated with hypromellose eyedrops, to severe keratitis with loss of visual acuity, acute glaucoma, or panophthalmitis (grade 3) or loss of vision (grade 4). Acute reactions in the ear are mild otitis media not requiring treatment (grade 1), moderate otitis media requiring topical medication (grade 2), severe otitis media with discharge (grade 3), and deafness (grade 4).

Late radiation toxicity is outside the scope of this chapter, but late reactions especially in the eye are exceedingly important and can include blindness from cataract or a dry eye from irradiation of the lacrimal gland, which are both treatable, to blindness and from retinal damage to optic nerve or chiasmal damage, which are permanent. Overdosage of radiation to spinal cord can result in paraplegia. Radiation tolerance doses for most organs are known with reasonable accuracy and for the anatomical structures within the eye in particular. Thus all radiation techniques around the head and neck are largely based on an underlying premise that the spinal cord and eye cannot be given more than the known tolerance doses.

ACUTE CANDIDIASIS

Acute candidiasis results from infection by yeasts of the Candida species, commonly by *C. albicans*. Candidal infections can occur in healthy persons in the mouth, pharynx, or genital tract, but in patients with HNSCC and especially if receiving radiotherapy, candidal infection is common. In immunocompromised patients, systemic candidiasis can occur.

Acute candidiasis causes discomfort in the mouth and is a cause of oral pain and pain on swallowing. It is characterized by white patches as mentioned earlier. It can be effectively treated with nystatin suspension or fluconazole tablets or

suspension. Occasionally, esophageal candidiasis can occur and cause esophageal pain. Fluconazole suspension will usually eradicate the condition except in immunocompromised persons (Figs. 5.5.8–5.5.10).

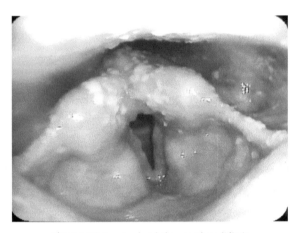

Figure 5.5.9 Laryngeal and pharyngeal candidiasis.

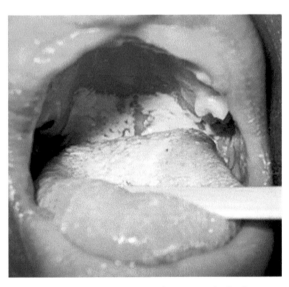

Figure 5.5.8 Oral candidiasis on the tongue and soft palate.

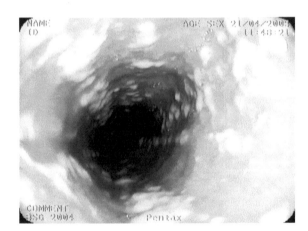

Figure 5.5.10 Esophageal candidiasis.

Index

Acute candidiasis, 98
Adenocarcinomas, 9–10
Adenoidal hypertrophy, 58–59
Adenoid cystic carcinoma, 9–10, 32, 51
Adenomas, 61, 74
Alcohol, 18
American Joint Committee on Cancer classification, 11
Amyloid, 60–61, 66
Apple core lesion, 49, 50
Atypical carcinoid, 32

Basal cephaloceles, 58
Benign goiter, 54
Benign nasopharyngeal tumors
    adenoidal hypertrophy, 58–59
    cephaloceles, 58
    chordomas, 58
    imaging investigation, 57
    juvenile nasal angiofibromas, 57
    pleomorphic adenomas, 58
    Rathke pouch, 58
    squamous papillomas, 57–58
    surgical treatment, 57
    symptoms, 57
Benign parapharyngeal tumors
    imaging investigations, 65
    neurogenic neoplasms
        neurofibromas, 64–65
        paragangliomas, 64–65
        schwannomas, 63–64
    salivary gland neoplasms, 63
    surgical management, 65
    symptoms, 65
Benign rhabdomyoma, 69
Benign tracheal tumors, 51
Betel nut, 18
Biopsy Forceps (Pentax), 1, 3
Buried flaps monitoring, 86–87

Cephaloceles, 58
Cervical lymphatics, 21–22
CHART. See Continuous hyperfractionated radiotherapy
Chemotherapy, 94
Chest x-ray, 52
Chondromas, 74
Chordomas, 58
Cicatricial pemphigoid, 70
Collagen, 78–79
Continuous hyperfractionated radiotherapy (CHART), 95
Cook–Swartz implantable Doppler, 86–87
Cricoid cartilage, 38
Cutaneous flaps monitoring, 86
Cysts
    epidermoid, 72

laryngeal, 72
mucus retention, 72
subglottic, 74

Direct phonoplasty, 78–79

Endolaryngeal laser surgery, 76–77
Endoscopic technique. See Transnasal laryngoesophagoscopy (TNLE)
ENT Flex Needle (Pentax), 1, 3
Epidermoid cysts, 72
Epithelial tumors, 60
Erythroplakia, 18
Esophageal candidiasis, 98
Esophageal pouch, 1
Esophageal tumors
    clinical appearance, 48–49
    epidemiology, 48
    histology, 48–49
    imaging investigations, 49
    surgical management, 49–50
    symptoms, 48
    TNM staging systems, 49
Esthesioneuroblastoma, 11
Ethmoid sinus cancer, 11–12

Failing flaps
    identification
        arterial insufficiency, 87–88
        intraoperative error, 87
        preoperative error, 87
        venous insufficiency, 88
    managing
        in free flaps, 89
        in pedicled flaps, 89
Fasciocutaneous free flaps, 85
Flap necrosis
    in free flaps, 89
    in pedicled flaps, 89
    signs of, 89
    treatment of, 89
Flaps
    definition, 82
    free
        fasciocutaneous, 85
        flap necrosis, 89
        monitoring of, 86
        muscle, 85
        musculocutaneous, 82–85
    pedicled, 82–85
        monitoring, 86

Gelfoam®, 15
Glottic tumors
    clinical appearance, 35

Glottic tumors (*Continued*)
    epidemiology, 35
    imaging systems, 36
    surgical management, 36–37
    symptoms, 35
    TNM staging systems, 36
Glottis
    cysts, 72
    granular cell tumors, 73
    granulomas, 72–73
    hyperkeratosis, 71
    nodules, 71–72
    papillomatosis, 71
    polyps, 71
    Reinke's edema, 72
Goiter, 54
Gracilis, 85
Granular cell tumors, 73
Granulomas, 72–73, 74

Head and neck squamous carcinoma (HNSCC)
    acute candidiasis, 98
    chemotherapy, 94
    radiotherapy
        radiation reactions, 95–98
        techniques and indications, 94–95
Hemangioma, 57, 62, 69
Hemangiomas, 74
HNSCC. *See* Head and neck squamous carcinoma
Hoarseness, 71
Hyperkeratosis, 71
Hypopharynx tumors
    clinical appearance, 41
    epidemiology, 40
    imaging investigations, 41
    surgical management, 41
    symptoms, 40
    TNM staging systems, 41

IMRT. *See* Intensity-modulated radiotherapy
111In-DTPA-D-Pheoctreotide, 11
Intensity-modulated radiotherapy (IMRT), 95

Juvenile nasal angiofibromas, 57
Juvenile nasopharyngeal angiofibroma (JNA), 13–14

Laryngeal candidiasis, 98
Laryngeal cysts, 72
Laryngectomy
    flap repair, 82
    primary repair, 82
Laryngoceles, 66
Laryngoscopy, 53
Leukoplakia, 18
Lichen planus, 18
Lignocaine, 4
Lingual thyroid, 61, 62
Lipomas, 68

Local anesthesia, 4, 7
Lymphatic spread, 26, 45
Lymphoma, 26

Malignant melanoma, 10
Maxillary sinus cancer, 11–12
Mediastinal leiomyosarcoma, 33
Mesenchymal tumors, 60
Minor salivary gland carcinomas, 23–25
Mucus retention cysts, 60, 72
Multinodular goiters, 54
Muscle-free flaps, 85
Musculocutaneous flaps, 82–85
Myocutaneous flaps monitoring, 86

Nasal cavity
    epidemiology, 10
    etiology, 8–9
    histology, 8–9
    imaging techniques, 10–11
    pathologic diagnosis, 11
    surgical management, 11–12
    symptoms, 8
    TNM staging system, 11–12
Nasopharyngeal angiofibroma, 17
Nasopharyngeal cancer (NPC), 13, 17
Nasopharynx
    anatomy, 13
    epidemiology, 13–15
    imaging examination, 15
    pathologic diagnosis, 15
    staging systems, 15
    surgical management, 15–17
Nd:YAG laser, 76
Neuroendocrine tumors, 66–67
Neurofibromas
    neurogenic neoplasms, 64–65
    supraglottis, 68
Neurogenic neoplasms
    neurofibromas, 64–65
    paragangliomas, 64–65
    schwannomas, 63–64
Non Hodgkin's lymphoma, 23–25
NPC. *See* Nasopharyngeal cancer

Octreoscan™, 11
Oncocytic cysts, 66
Oncocytomas, 66
Oral candidiasis, 98
Oral cavity
    at-risk sites, 18
    definition, 18
    examination, 18
    premalignant lesions, 18
    risk factors, 18
Oral squamous cell carcinoma
    clinical examination, 20–21
    dorsum of right side of tongue, 19

epidemiology, 20
five-year survival, 22
floor-of-the-mouth, 19
left lateral tongue, 19
right buccal and retromolar mucosa, 20
right buccal mucosa, 20
surgical management, 21–22
TNM staging system, 20
Oral submucous fibrosis, 18
Oropharynx tumors
clinical appearance, 23–24, 61
epidemiology, 23
imaging investigation, 61–62
imaging system, 24
staging system, 24
surgical management, 25, 62
symptoms, 60
Osteoradionecrosis, 21
Otalgia, 8

Papillomas, 61, 62
viral, 70
Papillomatosis, 71
Paragangliomas, 64–65
Paranasal sinuses
epidemiology, 10
etiology, 8–9
histology, 8–9
imaging techniques, 10–11
pathologic diagnosis, 11
surgical management, 11–12
symptoms, 8
TNM staging system, 11–12
Parapharyngeal space masses, 61
Parapharyngeal space tumors, 62
Parapharyngeal tumors, 63
Pectoralis major muscle, 82–83
Pedicled flaps
flap necrosis, 89
monitoring, 86
vs. musculocutaneous flaps, 82–85
Pentax Corporation, 1
Pharyngeal candidiasis, 98
Pharyngeal pouch, 2
Pharyngeal tonsils, 58
Pharyngocutaneous fistulae
early fistula formation, 90
late fistula formation, 90
Pleomorphic adenomas, 58, 61
Plummer–Vinson syndrome, 45
Polyps, 71
Portex®, 4
Post cricoid tumors
clinical appearance, 45
epidemiology, 45
histology, 45
imaging investigations, 45
staging systems
M staging, 46

N staging, 46
T staging, 45–46
surgical management, 47
symptoms, 45
Postcricoid web, 2
Pyriform fossa tumors
clinical apperance, 41, 42
epidemiology, 42
histopathology, 42
imaging investigations, 42–43
prognosis and outcomes, 44
surgical management
early cancer, 44
locally advanced cancer, 44
symptoms, 42
TNM staging systems, 44

Radiotherapy
radiation reactions, 95–98
techniques and indications, 94–95
Rathke pouch, 58
Recurrent laryngeal nerve (RLN), 54–55
Reinke's edema, 72
Retrosternal goiters, 55
Rhabdomyoma, 71
RLN. See Recurrent laryngeal nerve

Saccular cysts, 66
SCC. See Squamous cell carcinoma
Schwannomas
neurogenic neoplasms, 63–64
supraglottis, 67–68
Single solitary solid nodules, 54
Skin grafts, 22
Skin paddle flap method, 86
Skull base chordomas, 58
Squamous cell carcinoma (SCC)
nasal cavity, 8–10
oral
clinical examination, 20–21
dorsum of right side of tongue, 19
epidemiology, 20
five-year survival, 22
floor-of-the-mouth, 19
left lateral tongue, 19
right buccal and retromolar mucosa, 20
right buccal mucosa, 20
surgical management, 21–22
TNM staging system, 20
tongue base, 23–24
tonsil tumors, 26
Squamous papillomas, 57–58
Subglottic tumors
clinical appearance, 38
epidemiology, 38
imaging investigations, 38–39
surgical management, 39
symptoms, 38
TNM staging systems, 39

Subglottis
  adenomas, 74
  chondromas, 74
  cysts, 74
  granulomas, 74
  hemangiomas, 74
  systemic diseases, 74–75
Supraglottic tumors
  clinical appearance, 32
  epidemiology, 32
  imaging examination, 32–33
  surgical management, 34
  symptoms, 32
  TNM staging system, 33–34
Supraglottis
  amyloid, 66
  laryngoceles, 66
  lipomas, 68
  neuroendocrine tumors, 66–67
  neurofibromas, 68
  oncocytic cysts, 66
  oncocytomas, 66
  other tumors, 68–69
  saccular cysts, 66
  schwannomas, 67–68
Surgical management
  benign nasopharyngeal tumors, 57
  benign parapharyngeal tumors, 65
  esophageal tumors, 49–50
  glottic tumors, 36–37
  hypopharynx tumors, 41
  nasal cavity, 11–12
  nasopharynx, 15–17
  oral SCC, 21–22
  oropharynx tumors, 25
  paranasal sinuses, 11–12
  post cricoid tumors, 47
  pyriform fossa tumors, 44
  subglottic tumors, 39
  supraglottic tumors, 34
  thyroid tumors, 55
  tongue tumors, 31
  tonsil tumors, 27–28
  tracheal tumors, 53
Surgical voice restoration (SVR)
  benefits, 91
  for individual patients, 93
  long-term clinical management, 92–93
  tracheoesophageal puncture, 80
Swellings, 54
Systemic diseases, 74–75

Thornwaldt cyst, 58
Thyroid tumors
  clinical presentation, 54
  epidemiology, 54
  investigations, 54–55
  malignant tumors, 54
  prognosis, 56
  recurrent disease treatment, 56

surgical removal of thyroid gland, 55
surgical treatment, 55
TNLE. See Transnasal laryngoesophagoscopy
TNM staging systems
  base of tongue tumors, 29
  esophageal tumors, 49
  ethmoid sinus cancer, 11–12
  glottic tumors, 36
  hypopharynx tumors, 41
  maxillary sinus cancer, 11–12
  nasal cavity, 11–12
  nasopharyngeal cancer, 17
  oral SCC, 20
  paranasal sinuses, 11–12
  post cricoid tumors, 45–46
  pyriform fossa tumors, 44
  subglottic tumors, 39
  supraglottic tumors, 33–34
Tongue base SCC, 23–24
Tongue tumors
  clinical appearance, 29
  epidemiology, 29
  five-year survival rates, 31
  histology, 29
  imaging examination, 29
  surgical management, 31
  TNM staging system, 29
Tonsillar lymphomas, 26
Tonsil tumors
  clinical appearance, 26
  epidemiology
    lymphoma, 26
    squamous cell carcinomas, 26
  histopathology, 26
  imaging examination, 26–27
  prognosis and outcomes, 28
  surgical management
    early cancer, 27
    locally advanced cancer, 28
  T-staging system, 27
Tracheal tumors
  clinical appearance, 51–52
  epidemiology, 51
  histology, 51–52
  imaging investigations, 52–53
  surgical management, 53
  symptoms, 51
Tracheoesophageal puncture, 80–81
Transcricothyroid injection method, 78–79
Transnasal flexible endoscopy, 1
Transnasal laryngoesophagoscopy (TNLE)
  complications, 7
  direct phonoplasty, 78–79
  endolaryngeal laser surgery, 76–77
  esophageal pouch, 1
  local anesthesia, 4, 7
  location, 4
  vs. other endoscopic techniques, 7
  pain scores, 6–7
  position, 4

postcricoid web, 2
procedure, 4–5
recovery, 5
tracheoesophageal puncture, 80–81
Transoral laser surgery, 31
Trismus, 26
Tumor staging systems, 17

Verrucous carcinomas, 35
Viral papillomas, 70
Vocal cord medialization, 78–79
Vocal fold nodules, 71–72
Vocal fold polyps, 71

World Health Organization, 18

T - #0658 - 071024 - C116 - 246/189/5 [7] - CB - 9780415466301 - Gloss Lamination